Bounce

Back

Into

Shape

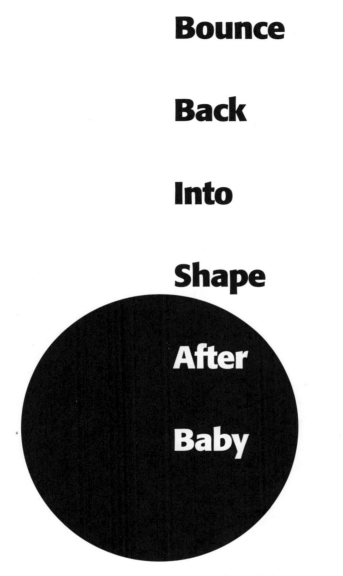

After

Baby

From One Mom
To Another

 Caroline Corning Creager, P. T.
Executive Physical Therapy Inc., Berthoud, Colorado

Executive Physical Therapy, Inc.
P.O. Box 1319
Berthoud, CO 80513
(970)532-2533
1-800-530-6878
email: Caroline@CarolineCreager.com
www.CarolineCreager.com

First Printing 2001

The author has made every effort to assure that the information in this book is accurate and current at the time of printing. The publisher and author take no responsibility for the use of the material in this book and cannot be held responsible for any typographical or other errors found. Please consult your physician before initiating this exercise program. The information in this book is not intended to replace medical advice.

ISBN: 0-9641153-5-2
Library of Congress Control Number: 2001129154

Cover Design by Kathy Tracy
Book Design by Kathy Tracy
Photographs by Geoffrey Wheeler (Chapters XII and XIII), Jill Creager (Chapters V, VII, IX, X, XI), and Robert Creager (Chapter II, V, VI, and XI)
Illustrations by Amy Brickey
Edited by Art Adams and Muriel E.Wheeler
Hair by Carol Woodard
Models: Christopher (white shirt), Michael (dark shirt), Caroline, and Robert Creager

About the Author:

Caroline Corning Creager, P.T.

Caroline Corning Creager is an award-winning author and an internationally recognized speaker on exercise topics. Caroline received her degree in Physical Therapy from the University of Montana. She is the C.E.O. of Executive Physical Therapy, Inc. in Colorado, U.S.A., and author of six books: *Bounce Back Into Shape After Baby*, *Therapeutic Exercises Using the Swiss Ball*, *Therapeutic Exercises Using Foam Rollers*, *Therapeutic Exercises Using Resistive Bands*, *Caroline Creager's Airobic Ball Strengthening Workout*, and *Caroline Creager's Airobic Ball Stretching Workout*.

She has written or been featured in numerous articles in: *WorldWideSpine*, *PhysioForum*, *Advance for PT's*, *Advance for OT's*, *OT/PT Today*, *Fitness*, *Cooking Light*, *Aspire*, and *Baby Steps*, and has been a guest speaker for the nationally televised, "America's Talking: Alive and Wellness", and for the Rehabilitation Training Network.

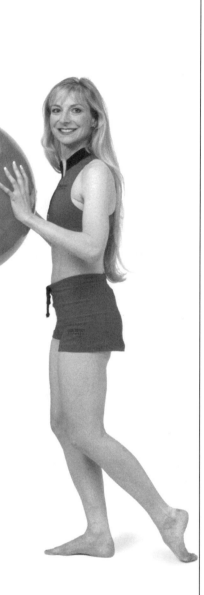

DEDICATIONS

To my husband, Robert, for being a wonderful father and a loving husband.

To my sons, Christopher Robert and Michael James, whose wet kisses and warm hugs have changed my life forever.

To my mother, Mary Corning, for being an inspiring and loving role model.

To my sister, Muriel (Beth) Wheeler, for being a part of my pregnancies, postpartum period, and sharing our special sister bond.

To my obstetrician, Dr. Carolyn Sue Schaffter, for helping me bring my boys into this world.

To my children's pediatrician, Dr. Nancy Greer, for her dedication and devotion to my children through the easy and more difficult times, and for taking the time to respect my concerns as a mother.

To my children's daycare provider, Irene Gilman and her husband Al, for being my boys' sunshine when it rained, and for giving me the time to make this book possible.

This Book Is Dedicated To All Mothers:

Mother

by Rachel Synder

Just one look and it's clear you're a mother.
Your cheeks have been stained with a mother's tears,
and your baby knows the sweet delight of a mother's kiss.
You move like a mother, standing in the grocery-store line and gently rocking side to side.
You kneel down in the grass to shade your baby from the sun.

You use a mother's language, radiating pride and joy
as you tell others of your baby's first word, first step, first tooth.
You have a mother's eyes, watching your little one grow more beautiful minute by minute.
And, of course, you also have a mother's touch, caressing your baby's skin
and soothing his baby fears.

You begin your day with a mother's prayer and end it with a mother's dreams.
You know there's no love like a mother's love, and no heart like the heart of a mother.
From head to toe, every day of the year, you're a mother, you're a woman.
You're you.

As seen in *American Baby*, May, 1999.
Reprinted with permission of the author.

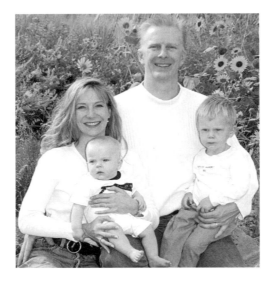

**In memory of my baby boy,
Gabriel Bliss Creager.**

Twin Angels, hearts entwined in Love
Two-flames that burned as one
Set forth in a tiny silver ship
New life! New light! The journey begun!

Yet all too soon, one light grew dim
And turned the ship back Home again
"I go no further, my brother, my friend,
For here my warrior's journey ends.
Please tell the others and please don't grieve,
For when Life is given, Life also receives."

Twin angels, souls entwined in Love
One shines below, one shines above
And in the brilliance of angel glow,
A mother's heart finds the courage to grow.

From Mom, Dad, big brother Christopher,
and twin brother Michael.

by Rachel Synder

PREFACE

This book is a treasure to me. It has given me an opportunity to capture a few precious moments in time with my children. The period of time after having your baby is oh so precious, challenging, and goes so quickly. For me, exercise during the post-partum period was a way to celebrate life with my boys, Christopher, and Michael, and share the loss of Michael's twin, Gabriel Bliss.

For you, I hope to share a fun and innovative way to exercise, so that you will make a life long commitment to exercise. And learn ways to take care of your abdomen, back, pelvic floor muscles, and posture, so you can feel good and enjoy this special time with your baby.

Including your children/family in your exercise program will give your children a jump-start on the importance of exercise in their daily life that will hopefully last them a lifetime too. By exercising with my sons, I believe I have made an early impact in their lives toward exercise. I remember a few of my son Christopher's first words, "Mommy, hold hand. Mommy Run. Let's Run." These few words make me so proud.

I am happy you are here to share my journey into motherhood, and exercise, and I hope your journey will be as fulfilling as mine. Enjoy.

Caroline

Caroline Corning Creager, P.T.

DONATION

Five percent of the sales of this book will be donated to the V.A.C.T.E.R.L. Foundation. The V.A.C.T.E.R.L. Foundation is a non-profit organization devoted to research, education, and providing financial assistance for rehabilitative equipment for children or adults that live with the challenges of V.A.T.E.R.S. or V.A.C.T.E.R.L.

The acronyms V.A.C.T.E.R.L. and V.A.T.E.R. were first coined to indicate a nonrandom association of birth anomalies that occur during the stage of organogenesis, or the first 4 weeks of after conception: **V**ertebral, **A**nal atresia, **T**racheo-**E**sophageal Fistula, **R**adial ray defects, and **R**enal anomalies. V.A.T.E.R.S. is a more antiquated term for V.A.C.T.E.R.L.

Contents

Contents, continued

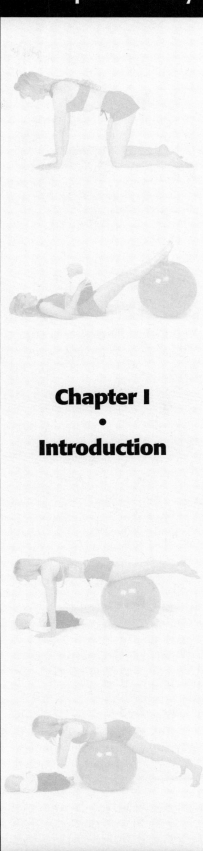

Chapter I
•
Introduction

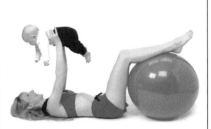

1.1 Baby Press

Good news: The Surgeon General's Report, 1996, states that "physical activity need not be strenuous to achieve health benefits. People who are usually inactive can improve their health and well-being by becoming even moderately active on a regular basis. Greater health benefits can be achieved by increasing the amount (duration, frequency, or intensity) of physical activity."

•

The American College of Sports Medicine (Med Sci Sports Exerc., 1998) also reports "many health benefits from physical activity can be achieved at lower intensities of exercise, if frequency and duration of training are increased appropriately. In this regard, physical activity can be accumulated through the day in shorter bouts of 10-minute durations."

Why Exercise?

Have you just had a baby? Are you exhausted and wondering how you can possibly find the time to fit in a workout? After I had my first son, Christopher, I was exhausted, just like you, and found that I had very little energy or time to work out.

I wanted to get back into shape as soon as possible, yet at my own pace and in the convenience of my own home. I also wanted my workout to be FUN, time and energy-efficient, and include my baby if possible (see photograph 1.1). Hence, I designed the *Bounce Back Into Shape After Baby* workouts.

I used this program after my first son was born, and I am following it a second time after the recent birth of my second child, Michael. Because my children and I have both enjoyed these fun-filled workouts so much, I decided to share them with you.

After you have had a baby, it becomes very difficult to find a block of time to do a 30–60 minute workout. I have found that on some days I may only have a 10-minute block of time to squeeze in a workout. Good news: The Surgeon General's Report, 1996, states that " physical activity need not be strenuous to achieve health benefits. People who are usually inactive can improve their health and well-being by becoming even moderately active on a regular basis. Greater health benefits can be achieved by increasing the amount [duration, frequency, or intensity] of physical activity."

Research at the University of Pittsburgh School of Medicine found that exercising in 10-minute time increments, several times a day, can be just as beneficial as working out for 30 minutes once a day. The American College of Sports Medicine (Med Sci Sports Exerc., 1998) also reports "many health benefits from physical activity can be achieved at lower intensities of exercise, if frequency and duration of training are increased appropriately. In this regard, physical activity can be accumulated through the day in shorter bouts of 10-minute durations."

This book is about FEELING GOOD about yourself, and spending quality time with your baby. When you feel good, weight loss will follow. Several studies have indicated that exercise significantly improves energy, and significantly decreases anxiety, depression, and mood disturbances (Koltyn, 1997, and Sampselle, 1999). Sampselle also found that 6 weeks after giving birth, the more active women had retained significantly less weight, 8.6 pounds (3.9 kilograms), and were more likely to participate in fun activities (socializing, hobbies, entertainment) than their less active counterparts. Clapp, 1998, found that one year after having a baby, women who exercise have three times less weight retention and two times less fat retention than women who don't exercise.

How this Book is Different

Keeping this in mind, I designed the *Bouncing Back Into Shape After Baby* mini-workouts to provide time-efficient 10-minute workouts, or less, that can be squeezed into any part of your day. These 10-minute workouts may be used one at a time or several at a time to make a 20 or 30-minute workout. The mini-workouts are located at the back of this book, and since the pages are perforated, you may tear them out, post them on a wall, or take them with you.

Bounce Back Into Shape After Baby focuses on strengthening your core abdominal, back, diaphragm, and pelvic floor (see illustration 1.2) muscles first, pages 31 – 58. As core strengthening is mastered, you may progress on to more dynamic exercises on the exercise ball, pages 100 – 162. These exercises use the principles learned throughout the beginning of this book, and provide more challenging levels of exercise due to the dynamic nature of the ball.

Whether you want to strengthen your pelvic floor muscles, tone your abdomen, or relieve tension in your lower back (see illustration 1.3 Low Back Stretch), this book provides balanced strengthening and stretching workouts that can be done in your own home. Each exercise page provides easy-to-read directions, illustrations, or photographs depicting how to do the exercise, and mini-workouts that are time and energy-efficient. The mini-workouts were designed to provide a variety of workouts for every level of fitness enthusiast – beginner to expert.

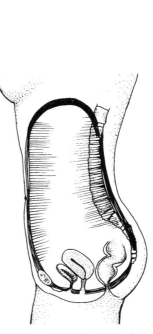

1.2 Core Stability Muscles

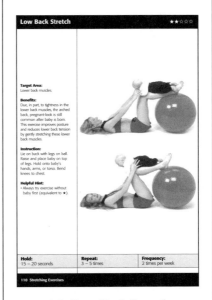

1.3 Low Back Stretch

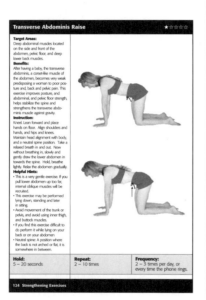

Transverse Abdominis Raise ★☆☆☆☆

Target Areas:
Deep abdominal muscles located on the side and front of the abdomen, pelvic floor, and deep lower back muscles.

Benefits:
After having a baby, the transverse abdominis, a corset-like muscle of the abdomen, becomes very weak predisposing a woman to poor posture and, back and pelvic pain. This exercise improves posture, and abdominal and pelvic floor strength, helps stabilize the spine and strengthens the transverse abdominis muscle against gravity.

Instruction:
Kneel. Lean forward and place hands on floor. Align shoulders and hands, and hips and knees. Maintain head alignment with body, and a neutral spine position. Take a relaxed breath in and out. Now without breathing in, slowly and gently draw the lower abdomen in towards the spine. Hold, breathe lightly. Relax the abdomen gradually.

Helpful Hints:
• This is a very gentle exercise. If you pull lower abdomen up too far, internal oblique muscles will be recruited.
• This exercise may be performed lying down, standing and later in sitting.
• Avoid movement of the trunk or pelvis, and avoid using inner thigh, and buttock muscles.
• If you find this exercise difficult to do perform it while lying on your back or on your abdomen.
• Neutral spine: A position where the back is not arched or flat, it is somewhere in between.

Hold:	Repeat:	Frequency:
5 – 20 seconds	2 – 10 times	2 – 3 times per day, or every time the phone rings.

124 Strengthening Exercises

1.4 Transverse Abdominis Raise

Starting a new exercise program, especially after having a baby, can be intimidating. For this reason, I have rated each exercise on a one to five star system. One star signifies the most basic exercise level, two stars – advanced beginner, three stars – intermediate, four stars – advanced, and five stars – expert. The star rating is located at the top of the page (see illustration 1.4). If the exercise received one star, then you would know right away that this exercise may be performed by a beginner, and a five star exercise means you may need to wait awhile before you try it, or that this exercise is for you if you are already in great shape.

This book is also unique in that it teaches you how to execute core strengthening techniques throughout the day. For these exercise principles to be successful, they must be carried through into activities of daily living at conscious and, after some time, unconscious levels, such as while lifting your baby in and out of a crib or car, holding your baby, or pushing your baby in a stroller.

A healthy and fit body does not come from exercising alone, so I have also covered *Scar Tissue Management Techniques, Demystifying Urinary and Fecal Incontinence, Look Like You Have Lost 10 Pounds by Improving Your Posture, Proper Body Mechanics for Lifting and Holding Your Baby, Breast-feeding and Exercise, and Introduction to the Ball.*

How to Use this Book

Bounce Back Into Shape After Baby provides general exercise guidelines and exercises that can be initiated within 24 hours after giving birth. Read the Exercise Guidelines After Vaginal Delivery, Chapter II, and Exercise Guidelines After Cesarean Delivery, Chapter III, first. These chapters cover how to begin, when not to exercise, how to monitor your body and adjust workouts depending on how your body feels, suggested workout routines, etc.

The exercises included in Chapter II and III are considered basic core strengthening exercises, because they focus on strengthening the muscles that provide support and stability to your pelvis, spine, and abdomen. During pregnancy, the abdomen, back, diaphragm, and pelvic floor muscles, become weak. For this reason, it is imperative to learn how to retrain and strengthen the core muscles before expanding a program to more advanced exercises that require a lot of support, strength, and stability, such as running, high impact aerobics, and three to five star ball exercises.

Core Strengthening exercises as illustrated in Chapter V will focus on the working relationship of the abdominal, back, diaphragm, and pelvic floor muscles. Mini-workouts are also provided to focus on each of these areas of the body. After you have become proficient at performing the core strengthening exercises (this may take 2 to 6 weeks depending on your current physical capability) you may progress on to higher level exercises, such as aerobic and ball exercises (Chapters X to XIII). A good rule of thumb is, if you can sit on a ball comfortably and you are able to perform the core strengthening exercises – then you are most likely ready to begin ball exercises.

The Mini-Workouts, Chapter XIV, are designed as a quick reference to the exercises illustrated throughout the book, and to give you workout routine ideas (see illustration 1.5). The suggested workouts add variety to the workout, and provide greater strength and endurance gains in less time.

Interspersed throughout the aforementioned chapters, I have included information that is relevant to the postpartum period and may influence your exercise directly or indirectly. These chapters include Scar Tissue Management (Chapter IV), Incontinence (Chapter VI), Posture (Chapter VII), Body Mechanics (Chapter VIII), and Breast-feeding (Chapter IX).

Congratulations on becoming a new mother! I hope you enjoy this book and have fun as you *Bounce Back Into Shape After Baby*.

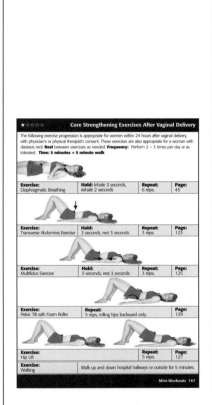

1.5 Mini-Workout

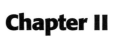

Chapter II
•
Vaginal Delivery and Exercise Guidelines

Women who are attended to by a midwife are more likely to have a vaginal delivery and are less likely to have surgical incisions, such as with a cesarean section or an episiotomy (Gerrits et. al, 1994, Robinson et. al, 2000).

•

It is estimated that between 50–90 percent of women will have an episiotomy (Hordnes, 1994).

•

Women who receive midline episiotomies are 4.2 to 12 (younger women vs. older women) times more likely to experience a rupture of the anal sphincter than women who receive mediolateral incisions (Shiono et. al., 1990).

Vaginal Delivery

The majority of women throughout the world deliver their babies vaginally as opposed to a cesarean delivery. Women in the Netherlands are most likely, more than 90%, to delivery their babies vaginally, while Chinese and Latin American women are least likely, less than 50% (Noble, 1998 and Qian, 2001). Women who are attended to by a midwife are more likely to have a vaginal delivery and are less likely to have surgical incisions, such as with a cesarean section or an episiotomy (Gerrits, et. al, 1994, Robinson, et. al, 2000).

Vaginal delivery, without an episiotomy or perineal (the area between the vagina and rectum) tear, is ideal. It typically decreases trauma to the pelvic floor muscles leading to less discomfort in the perineum, and a more rapid return to exercise and sexual intercourse (Signorello, et. al., 2001). Eason and Feldman (2000), recommend preventing perineal trauma during childbirth by avoiding episiotomy and forceps deliveries and slowing delivery of the head to allow the perineum time to stretch. Integrity of the perineum was best among clinicians who had the lowest episiotomy rates (Low, et. al., 2000).

The country in which you reside, or your doctor's personal preference toward episiotomies, greatly influences the chance of delivering your baby with or without an episiotomy (Robinson et. al., 2000, Scott-Wright, et. al., 1999). For these reasons, episiotomy rates vary greatly. It is estimated that between 50–90 percent of women will have an episiotomy (Hordnes, 1994). First time mothers receive episiotomies more frequently than mothers who have delivered more than one baby.

The presumed benefits of an episiotomy are prevention of perineal lacerations, pelvic floor damage, and release of harmful pressure on the head of the baby. Hordnes reports there is very little evidence to substantiate these findings. On the contrary, many studies have shown that high episiotomy rates are associated with an increased risk for perineal lacerations, especially ruptures of the anal sphincter.

Perez indicates that an episiotomy is necessary when a woman's baby must be delivered due to bradycardia, a very slow heart rate (Perez, 2001). This was the case for my first son's delivery. I had wanted to deliver my baby without an episiotomy. However, after my son's heart rate steadily plunged, I was given a mid-line episiotomy. I fortunately had no complications from the episiotomy, and delivered a healthy baby boy.

Women who receive midline episiotomies are 4.2 to 12 (younger women vs. older women) times more likely to experience a rupture of the anal sphincter than women who receive mediolateral incisions (Shiono, et. al., 1990). A midline incision is made from the vagina back toward the anus, and the mediolateral incision is made diagonally out away from the vagina (see illustration 2.1).

There are pros and cons for both types of episiotomies. As mentioned, there is less chance of an anal sphincter rupture with a mediolateral incision (de Leeuw, et. al., 2001), however, there is typically more discomfort, greater scar tissue involvement, and more trauma to the pelvic floor muscles. A midline episiotomy increases your chance of an anal sphincter rupture, yet decreases the trauma to the pelvic floor muscles (if the perineum does not tear) and consequently heals quicker with less scar tissue.

Women who require that their babies be delivered by forceps have almost twice the risk of perineal trauma leading to fecal incontinence as compared to women delivering their baby by vacuum extraction (MacArthur, 2001). Women who have had either of these procedures typically experience more discomfort during intercourse (Signorello, et. al., 2001) and take longer to heal, leading potentially to more scar tissue production.

Scar tissue management of an episiotomy scar or tear of the perineum, is often overlooked. Scar tissue massage should be initiated 5 – 8 days after giving birth. Please refer to the chapter on Scar Tissue Management Techniques, page 24.

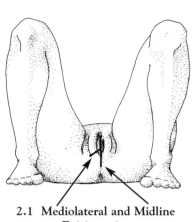

2.1 Mediolateral and Midline Episiotomies

If you have swelling, discomfort, or pain in the area of the perineum, **R.I.C.E.** it with **T**.

Rest
Ice
Compress
Elevate
and
Toilet Training Techniques

Be sure to rest as frequently as possible. Ice the perineal area within the 36 hours following childbirth, and use ice or heat after that time. A frozen bag of peas, wrapped in a towel, conforms to this area nicely. Lightly compress the area by wearing a comfortable pair of panties, lined with a sanitary pad. Elevate your feet, legs, and bottom with pillows. Your feet should be the most elevated, followed by the legs, and bottom. Follow the Toilet Training Techniques as outlined on page 63.

You may wonder how a vaginal, cesarean, forceps, vacuum, or episiotomy delivery is relevant to exercise? All of these factors, your body type, general fitness level, the rate your body heals, and level of motivation influence your desire and/or ability to begin exercising.

It will take time before you can return to the same exercise intensity that you enjoyed before pregnancy. YOUR EXERCISE ROUTINES SHOULD BE RESUMED GRADUALLY AND PACED TO ACCOMMODATE YOUR PHYSICAL CAPABILITY (ACOG, 1994. No 189).

I have designed an exercise regimen I recommend you begin within 24 hours after giving birth to your beautiful baby. This program can be found on page 14.

Many of the physiological changes of pregnancy persist for four to six weeks after the baby is delivered. The heart beats faster, the joints are more lax, the body fatigues faster, and hormones levels are normalizing. It will take time before you can return to the same exercise intensity that you enjoyed before pregnancy. YOUR EXERCISE ROUTINES SHOULD BE RESUMED GRADUALLY AND PACED TO ACCOMMODATE YOUR PHYSICAL CAPABILITY (ACOG, 1994. No 189).

Dr. Clapp reported that 40% of the women he studied (these women exercised before and during their pregnancies) returned to regular exercise in the first two weeks after the birth of their baby and exercised at a light to moderate intensity.

Keeping this in mind, more intense exercise, such as jogging, aerobics, and 4 – 5 star ball exercises (as seen on the top of each exercise page), may be initiated when you feel up to it, or as recommended by your physician. Dr. James Clapp, a renowned researcher on pregnancy, exercise, and the post-partum period, has come to this conclusion after extensive research on when to begin exercise after giving birth: "If it doesn't hurt or cause the woman to bleed heavily, it's OK." He further reports, "in most instances, women who continue exercise throughout pregnancy and begin again shortly after the birth do not experience pain; instead, they reap multiple emotional and physical benefits without compromising breast, bladder, or sexual function."

"NO PAIN NO GAIN" IS A MYTH. Pain is your body's way of telling you that something is not quite right.

Body size, shape, body awareness, type of delivery, etc. can influence your ability to perform an exercise.

Dr. Clapp (1998) reported that 40% of the women he studied (these women exercised before and during their pregnancies) returned to regular exercise in the first two weeks after the birth of their babies and exercised at a light to moderate intensity. He also found that stress incontinence (loss of urine with coughing, lifting, etc.) that was evident after childbirth, lasted less than one month in the exercise group, versus three months to a year in the non-exercise group.

One of the best pieces of advice I can share with you is to LISTEN TO YOUR BODY! If exercise feels good, and you are enjoying what you do, then LISTEN TO YOUR BODY and continue doing what you are doing. If you are having discomfort or pain with a specific type of exercise, then you need to LISTEN TO YOUR BODY as well.

"NO PAIN NO GAIN" IS A MYTH. Pain is your body's way of telling you that something is not quite right Pain will usually lead to swelling, soreness, and more pain. Try a different exercise, reduce your exercise repetitions, frequency, or stop performing this particular exercise until you can perform it without pain or discomfort.

Many times women get caught up in the QUANTITY of exercises they perform. How many situps can you do? The key is really the QUALITY of movement while performing the exercise. Ask instead, did that exercise make you feel good? Remember QUALITY NOT QUANTITY.

When your body begins to fatigue, it causes you to substitute, or use the incorrect muscles to perform an exercise. For instance, if you are performing the Kegel exercise on page 52, and you are able to perform 3 repetitions before fatigue, and on the fourth repetition you begin to squeeze your buttocks and thighs and clench your jaw, then it is time to stop. Relax and remember, FATIGUE CAUSES MUSCLE SUBSTITUTION.

Body size, shape, body awareness, type of delivery, etc. can influence your ability to perform an exercise. For example, if you find it difficult to perform the Transverse Abdominis exercise while lying on your back, page 123, try doing the exercise while you are on your hands and knees, page 124. Or if you are having a difficult time performing a Pushup on the ball, try a Baby Press-Up instead. If Kegel exercises, page 52, are becoming easy to do, and you find you are in great shape, try performing a Standing Squat to Heel Raises while you contract your pelvic floor muscles, page 162. ADAPT THE EXERCISE TO YOUR BODY, NOT YOUR BODY TO THE EXERCISE.

7 Tips to a Successful Exercise Program

1. Your exercise routines should be resumed gradually and paced to accommodate your physical capability.

2. Listen to your body.

3. "No pain, no gain" is a myth.

4. Quality not quantity.

5. Fatigue causes muscle substitution.

6. Adapt the exercise to your body, not your body to the exercise.

7. Customize your exercise program to meet the individualized needs of your own body.

   - Caroline C. Creager

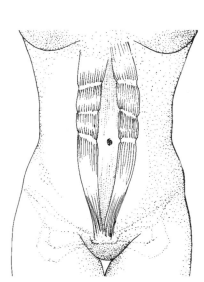

2.2 Diastasis Recti

If you had a difficult delivery or even if you had a wonderful delivery, it may take you more or less time to *Bounce Back Into Shape After Baby*. CUSTOMIZE YOUR EXERCISE PROGRAM TO MEET THE INDIVIDUALIZED NEEDS OF YOUR OWN BODY.

A well-rounded exercise program includes stretching, strengthening, and aerobic exercises. Please read chapters XII, XIII, and X respectively for more information on these different types of exercise. Begin with the exercises depicted in this chapter and core strengthening exercises as recommended on pages 37, 42, and 58, and then progress to aerobic, and ball stretching and strengthening exercises. Follow the 7 TIPS TO A SUCCESSFUL EXERCISE PROGRAM and GENERAL EXERCISE GUIDELINES AFTER A VAGINAL DELIVERY, and enjoy your exercise journey.

General Exercise Guidelines After Vaginal Delivery

1. You may begin the recommended exercises on page 14, within twenty-four hours after giving birth, with a physician's or healthcare professional's consent.

2. If you have had a cesarean birth, please refer to the cesarean exercise guidelines.

3. Determine if you have a separation of your abdominal muscles, diastasis recti (see illustration 2.2), by following the directions on page 39. If you find that you do have a diastasis recti, then follow the exercises as directed on page 40 before you begin performing a more advanced exercise program or do any heavy lifting.

4. If at any time you experience bright red or increased vaginal bleeding, pain, weakness, or dizziness with exercise, stop. Revise your exercise regimen by reducing intensity, frequency, duration, and/or type of exercise. If any of these symptoms persist with exercise, please contact your physician.

5. If you have a breast, vaginal, or incision site (episiotomy) infection, please contact your obstetrician before initiating or continuing your exercise regimen.

6. If you can sit on a ball comfortably and you are able to perform the core strengthening exercises – then you are most likely ready to begin ball exercises (see illustration 2.3). Avoid bouncing motions on the ball until 4 weeks after giving birth, or until the bouncing motion does not cause any discomfort in the pelvic floor, abdominal, or back region. Bouncing on the ball should be performed only if you are continent of urine.

7. Six weeks after having your baby, you may gradually resume your pre-pregnancy exercise routine. Pace yourself to accommodate your current physical capability (Exercise During Pregnancy and the Postpartum Period, ACOG, 1994. No 189).

8. Previously sedentary people who begin physical activity programs should start with a short session (5 – 10 minutes) of physical activity and gradually build up to a desired level of activity *(Physical Activity and Health: A Report of the Surgeon General)*.

9. Women with chronic health problems, such as heart disease, diabetes, or obesity, or who are at risk for these conditions should first consult a physician before beginning a new program of physical activity *(Physical Activity and Health: A Report of the Surgeon General)*.

10. Drink lots of water. Drink a minimum of 10 glasses of water a day, and even more if you exercise and breast-feed.

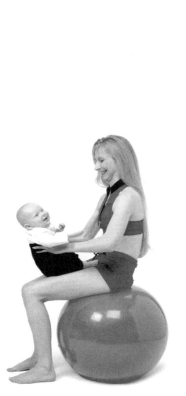

2.3 Pelvic Tilt while Sitting on Ball with Baby

The following exercise progression is appropriate for a woman within 24 hours after a vaginal delivery, with a physician's or physical therapist's consent. These exercises are also appropriate for a woman with diastasis recti. **Rest** between exercises as needed. **Frequency:** Perform 2 – 3 times per day or as tolerated.

Time: 5 minutes + 5 minute walk

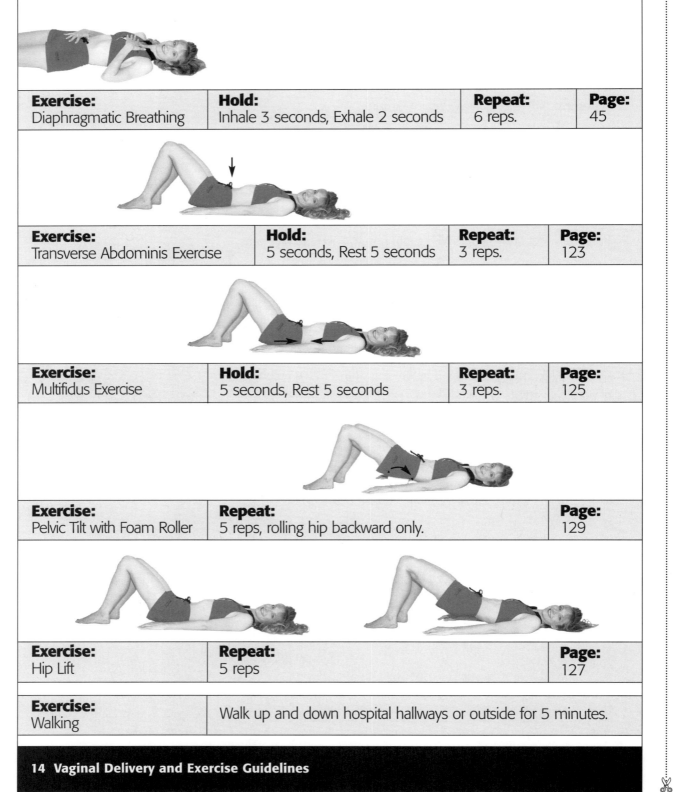

Exercise:	Hold:	Repeat:	Page:
Diaphragmatic Breathing	Inhale 3 seconds, Exhale 2 seconds	6 reps.	45

Exercise:	Hold:	Repeat:	Page:
Transverse Abdominis Exercise	5 seconds, Rest 5 seconds	3 reps.	123

Exercise:	Hold:	Repeat:	Page:
Multifidus Exercise	5 seconds, Rest 5 seconds	3 reps.	125

Exercise:	Repeat:	Page:
Pelvic Tilt with Foam Roller	5 reps, rolling hip backward only.	129

Exercise:	Repeat:	Page:
Hip Lift	5 reps	127

Exercise:	
Walking	Walk up and down hospital hallways or outside for 5 minutes.

Chapter III

•

Cesarean Delivery and Exercise Guidelines

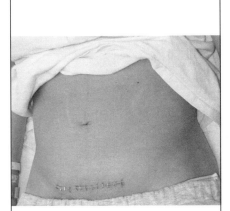

3.1 Cesarean Incision

Thirty-one percent of African American women and twenty-one percent of Caucasian women in the U.S., have had cesarean births (Scott-Wright, et. al,. 1999).

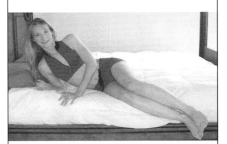

3.2 Log Roll

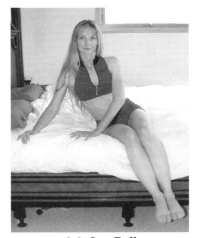

3.3 Log Roll

Cesarean Delivery

Cesarean refers to the ancient story of how Caesar or an ancestor of his had been born by cutting through the mother's abdominal and uterine walls to deliver the child. (*Webster's New World Dictionary*). More often than not, a cesarean birth is downplayed in our society as being "minor surgery".

As a physical therapist, I routinely asked my clients, "have you had any type of surgery?" If a woman's response was, "Yes, I had a cesarean section," I would unconsciously categorize this as a "minor type of surgery." My second child, Michael, was born by cesarean due to his breech position and cardiac problems. Now I know better than to assume that just because cesarean births are common, (31% of African-American and 21% of Caucasian births in the U.S. were by cesarean (Scott-Wright, et. al., 1999)), that this type of surgery is minor. I will never make that mistake again.

In order for a child to be born by cesarean, the obstetrician must cut through the following layers: skin, connective tissue, abdominal muscles (usually these muscles are moved aside), and wall of the uterus (see illustration 3.1). The surgeon must then pull to get the baby out, causing additional soreness and bruising. No wonder you are very sore and have difficulty getting in and out of bed, standing up straight, and walking.

To eliminate pain and discomfort involved with getting in and out of bed, it is best to learn how to log roll. A log roll is a technique designed to decrease pressure and tension on your abdominal incision and back by rolling as a unit to your side. To implement a log roll as depicted (see illustrations 3.2 and 3.3). Lie on your back. Bend your knees by drawing one knee up at a time. Roll to your side as a unit, keeping your knees together. Place your elbow and your other hand on the bed. Push up with elbow and hand, as you lower your feet off the bed. Keep pushing until you are in a sitting position. To get into bed, follow the same technique, but reversed.

Be careful not to move too much during the first few days after a c-section. I did just this, and caused a hematoma, a blood clot, to form under the incision. Unfortunately, the hematoma caused additional scar tissue adhesion, and my hematoma took many months to heal. Massaging the area of the scar with a hematoma is not recommended because you run the risk of exacerbating the hematoma. Follow the R.I.C.E. it with T. guidelines for reducing swelling, discomfort, or pain in the abdominal area.

Exercises or scar tissue massage that pull on this fragile scar tissue are not recommended during the first 5 to 8 days after your cesarean. However, scar tissue massage is recommended and you may begin as soon as the incision has healed and staples are removed. Please refer to the chapter on Scar Tissue Management Techniques.

Walking is an excellent form of exercise that may be performed during these first 5 to 8 days and you may also begin modified exercises within several days after a cesarean delivery with your physician's consent. The gentle pumping action of your muscles promotes healing by improving circulation and reducing swelling in the area of the incision.

I recommend you work on diaphragmatic breathing, sitting/standing up straight, and Exercises After Cesarean Delivery, as outlined on pages 20 – 21, and read in more detail about the 7 Tips to a Successful Exercise Program. For higher level exercises, many physicians recommend you begin exercising between 4 to 6 weeks after delivery, or as Dr. James Clapp states "if (exercise makes you) hurt, stop, and if it feels good, it's probably OK."

7 Tips to a Successful Exercise Program

1. Your exercise routines should be resumed gradually and paced to accommodate your physical capability.
2. Listen to your body.
3. "No pain, no gain" is a myth.
4. Quality not quantity.
5. Fatigue causes muscle substitution.
6. Adapt the exercise to your body, not your body to the exercise.
7. Customize your exercise program to meet the individualized needs of your own body.

-Caroline C. Creager

.

If you have swelling, discomfort, or pain in the abdominal area, **R.I.C.E**. it with **T**.

Rest
Ice
Compress
Elevate
and
Toilet Training Techniques

Be sure to rest as frequently as possible. Ice the abdominal area within the 36 hours following surgery, and use ice or heat after that time. Lightly compress and support your abdomen with a pillow when coughing, or vomiting. Elevate your feet, legs, and bottom with pillows. Your feet should be the most elevated, followed by the legs, and bottom. Follow the Toilet Training Techniques as outlined on page 63.

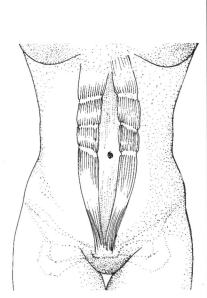

3.4 Diastasis Recti

General Exercise Guidelines After Cesarean Delivery

1. Within twenty-four hours after giving birth by cesarean, you may begin exercises as recommended on page 20 with a physician's or healthcare professional's consent.

2. If at any time you experience bright red or increased vaginal bleeding, pain, weakness, or dizziness with exercise, stop. Revise your exercise regimen by reducing intensity, frequency, duration, and/or type of exercise. If any of these symptoms persist with exercise, please contact your healthcare professional.

3. Determine if you have a separation of your abdominal muscles, diastasis recti, by following the directions on page 39. If you find that you do have a diastasis recti, then follow the exercises as directed on page 40 before you perform a more advanced exercise program or do any heavy lifting.

4. Initially, when doing the Abdominal and Back Stretch on page 108, do only one repetition of the stretch. Increase the number of stretches gradually. There should not be any discomfort, heat, redness, swelling, or lingering soreness in the area of your scar after stretching. If you experience any of these symptoms after stretching, stop. Give your incision a few more days to heal and then try again.

5. If you can sit on a ball comfortably and you are able to perform the core strengthening exercises – then you are most likely ready to begin ball exercises (see illustration 3.5). Avoid bouncing motions on the ball until 4 weeks after giving birth, or until the bouncing motion does not cause any discomfort in the pelvic floor, abdominal, or back region. Bouncing on the ball should be performed only if you are continent of urine.

6. If you have a breast, vaginal, or incision site infection, please contact your obstetrician before initiating or continuing your exercise regimen.

7. Six weeks after having your baby, you may gradually resume your pre-pregnancy exercise routine. Pace yourself to accommodate your current physical capability (Exercise During Pregnancy and the Postpartum Period, ACOG, 1994. No 189).

8. Previously sedentary people who begin physical activity programs should start with short sessions (5–10 minutes) of physical activity and gradually build up to a desired level of activity (*Physical Activity and Health: A Report of the Surgeon General*).

9. Women with chronic health problems, such as heart disease, diabetes, or obesity, or who are at risk for these conditions should first consult a physician before beginning a new program of physical activity (*Physical Activity and Health: A Report of the Surgeon General*).

10. Drink lots of water. Drink a minimum of 10 glasses of water a day, and even more if you exercise and breast-feed.

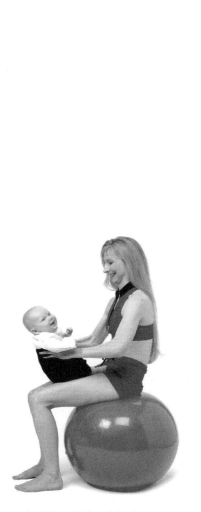

3.5 Pelvic Tilt while Sitting on Ball with Baby

Core Strengthening Exercise Progression After Cesarean Delivery ★☆☆☆☆

The following exercise progression is appropriate for a woman within 24 hours after a cesarean delivery with a physician's or physical therapist's consent. These exercises are also appropriate for a woman with diastasis recti. **Rest** between exercises as needed. **Frequency:** Perform 2 - 3 times per day or as tolerated.

Time: 5 minutes + 5 minute walk

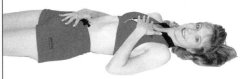

Exercise: Diaphragmatic Breathing	**Hold:** Inhale 3 seconds, Exhale 3 seconds	**Repeat:** 6 reps.	**Page:** 45

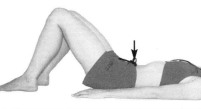

Exercise: Transverse Abdominis Exercise	**Hold:** 5 seconds, Rest 5 seconds	**Repeat:** 3 reps.	**Page:** 123

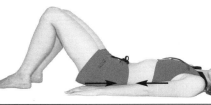

Exercise: Multifidus Exercise	**Hold:** 5 seconds, Rest 5 seconds	**Repeat:** 3 reps.	**Page:** 125

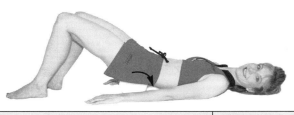

Exercise: Pelvic Tilt with Foam Roller	**Repeat:** 5 reps, rolling hip backward only.	**Page:** 129

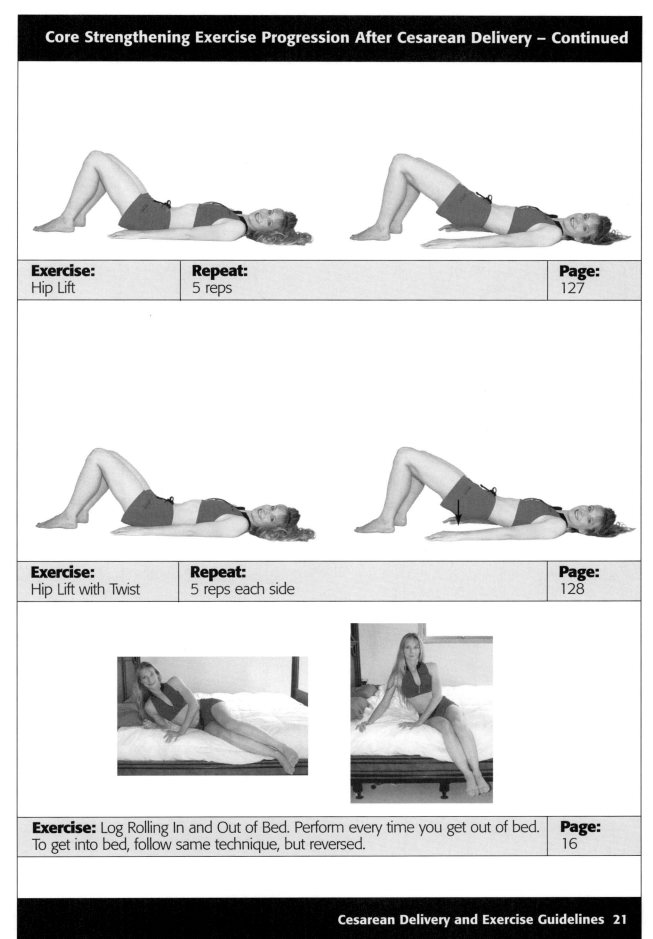

Exercise: Hip Lift	**Repeat:** 5 reps	**Page:** 127

Exercise: Hip Lift with Twist	**Repeat:** 5 reps each side	**Page:** 128

Exercise: Log Rolling In and Out of Bed. Perform every time you get out of bed. To get into bed, follow same technique, but reversed.	**Page:** 16

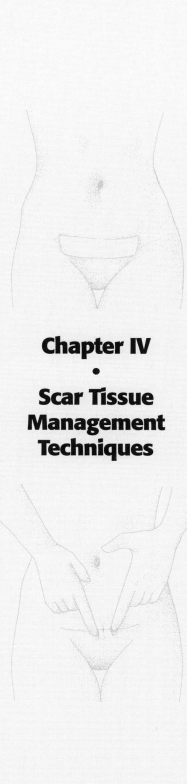

Chapter IV
·
Scar Tissue Management Techniques

To be most effective, scar tissue massage should occur within the first 14 weeks (Cummings and Reynolds, 1998) after your cesarean or episiotomy.

•

Resting the abdominal region, and preventing movements that pull on the scar for the first 5 to 8 days after your cesarean, is essential for the healing process of the scar.

•

At 5 to 8 days after your cesarean section, the scar has strengthened enough, via collagen fibers, to permit removal of your staples and/or sutures.

Introduction to Scar Tissue Management Techniques

One of the most over-looked areas of the body after giving birth is the incision site from an episiotomy or cesarean section. The visible portion of the incision will typically heal without incident, however scar tissue adhesion (thickened tissue) frequently occur underneath the visible scar.

If the scar tissue adhesion are not broken up early on, these adhesion may cause the scar to become thick, tender to touch, and less pliable. Thick and less pliable scar tissue may cause areas of the scar to become stuck or lumpy. To find out if you have areas that are stuck, refer to "Is My Scar Stuck?" on page 27.

What is the best way to prevent scar tissue adhesion? The best way is to gently massage the scar. To be most effective, scar tissue massage should occur within the first 14 weeks (Cummings and Reynolds, 1998) after your cesarean or episiotomy.

New scar formation is very fragile the first few days, and pink in color due to increased blood flow to the area. It takes at least two days for collagen fibers to begin binding the scar tissue together. Resting the abdominal region, and preventing movements that pull on the scar for the first 5 to 8 days after your cesarean, is essential for the healing process of the scar. Walking and other gentle forms of exercise are beneficial and appropriate during this time period.

At 5 to 8 days after your cesarean section, the scar has strengthened enough, via collagen fibers, to permit removal of your staples and/or sutures. It is at this time, or when the scab formation has fallen off, that you would want to begin massaging your scar. Follow the 7 Steps to Successful Episiotomy and Cesarean Scar Tissue Management, on pages 27 – 29.

Can you still massage your scar even though it has been more than 14 weeks since your episiotomy or cesarean section? Yes, you may begin using the massage techniques as listed below at any time. These techniques, as mentioned previously, are more successful in preventing scar tissue adhesion if performed within the first 14 weeks after surgery. If you find you already have scar tissue adhesion, you may need a more aggressive form of scar tissue management to break it up.

If after 2 to 4 weeks of massaging your scar, you continue to feel areas of the scar that are stuck, you may want to contact a physical therapist or other trained healthcare professional to assist you with a deeper form of scar tissue massage, such as myofascial release or visceral manipulation.

Myofascial release, visceral manipulation, and/or ultrasound can be used in conjunction with scar massage to break up scar tissue adhesion. These techniques require the expertise of a healthcare practitioner such as a physical therapist, or Doctor of Osteopathic Medicine (DO). Please contact your healthcare professional to learn more about how ultrasound, myofascial release and/or visceral manipulation can assist with breaking up your scar tissue adhesion. The majority of physical therapy clinics and physicians' offices are equipped with an ultrasound machine. To find a healthcare professional who practices myofascial release in your area, you may call Myofascial Treatment Centers at (800) FASCIAL or visit their website at www.myofascialrelease.com and/or The Upledger Institute for visceral manipulation at www.upledger.com or (800) 233-5880.

For optimal scar tissue management and prevention of these problems, follow the guidelines outlined in this chapter and follow up with pelvic floor and back strengthening exercises as outlined in Chapter V.

When is scar tissue massage not recommended?
1. During the first 5 to 8 days after surgery.
2. If you have an infection.
3. If you have a blood clot or disorder of the blood.
4. If you are pregnant.
5. If you have pre-cancerous or malignant lesions present.

When will my scar color change from a pink color to gray/white?
It may take up to one year or more for a scar to mature, or lose its pink color. As the scar begins to mature it will lose some blood vessels to the area, causing the scar to turn gray/white.

•

How will scar tissue adhesion affect you if you do not massage the scar?
Scar tissue adhesion, along with weak abdominal, and mid-back muscles, may contribute to pelvic pain, poor posture, and mid and low back pain.

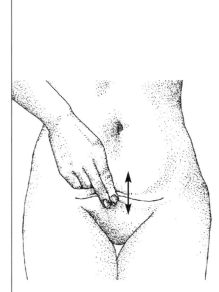

4.1 Friction Massage. Use very light pressure, approximately 2 to 3 ounces (60–90 grams).

The following massage tips were designed as a quick reference and to facilitate the success of your scar tissue management.

Scar Tissue Massage Tips

1. Begin gentle massage of scar tissue after suture/staple removal, and scab formation has fallen off, usually on day 5 to 8.

2. Massage to tolerance. Begin with only 2 to 5 minutes of massage, and progress to 10 to 15 minutes unless otherwise noted.

3. Avoid using lotion or oil with these massage techniques. (A slick surface, as caused by lotion or oil, causes the fingers to slip back and forth over the scar. It is important to AVOID sliding your fingers across the skin. Your fingers should MOVE WITH THE SCAR).

4. When performing massage, use very light pressure, approximately 2 to 3 ounces (60–90 grams)

5. Stretch in the direction of greatest restriction unless otherwise directed.

6. Massage/knead the muscles and tissue surrounding your scar.

7. If you find scar tissue massage to be uncomfortable, try massaging your scar after taking a bath or shower. Since warm tissue moves more easily than cold tissue, be cautious not to massage the area too much.

8. If your scar remains adhered even after massaging it, you may be a candidate for myofascial release or visceral manipulation. Contact your local physical therapist or Doctor of Osteopathic Medicine (DO).

9. Talk to your local healthcare professional about how ultrasound may help prevent or reduce your scar tissue adhesion. If a healthcare professional uses ultrasound in the abdominal area, make sure the ultrasound is not applied over the ovaries.

7 Steps to Successful Episiotomy and Cesarean Scar Tissue Management

1) **Is My Scar Stuck?:** Test your scar to determine if you have any areas of the scar that are "stuck" to underlying tissue. Place your thumb and index finger on opposite ends of scar. Gently try and push your thumb and finger together. If your scar and skin make a rounded arch (see illustration 4.2) out away from your body, then outer layers of scar tissue are not adhered. If the scar looks more similar to an "M" with the center of the scar stuck and an arch formation on either side (see illustration 4.3), then you have scar tissue adhesion present. If you are unable to lift the scar in any fashion away from your body, then you have many areas of scar tissue adhesion or the tissue may still be swollen from surgery.

2) **Scar Desensitization:** If you find your scar is sensitive to touch, you may find that you will need to desensitize it before you begin massage. Place a wet washcloth, or dry washcloth if tolerated, over the scar and lightly rub it. Continue rubbing the scar with a wet/dry washcloth for 1 - 2 minutes, or as tolerated. Once you are able to touch your scar without difficulty, progress to massaging it, or try scar tissue taping as in step 7.

3) **Up, Down, & Side Glide:** Place two fingers perpendicular to the top of your scar. Gently press the scar toward your right side. Avoid sliding your fingers across the skin. Your fingers should MOVE WITH THE SCAR. By moving with your scar, you enable it to be separated from tissue that lies beneath it. USE VERY LIGHT PRESSURE, APPROX. 2 - 3 OUNCES. When the skin stops moving, continue to hold light pressure on the scar for 1 to 2 minutes. Slowly raise your fingers off the scar. This technique may feel uncomfortable, but will subside with time. Now pull the scar toward opposite side, hold 1 - 2 minutes. Repeat, lightly pushing the scar up toward your head, and pulling it down toward your feet (see illustration 4.1). You will typically find one direction is more STUCK than another. Spend more time going in the direction that feels stuck.

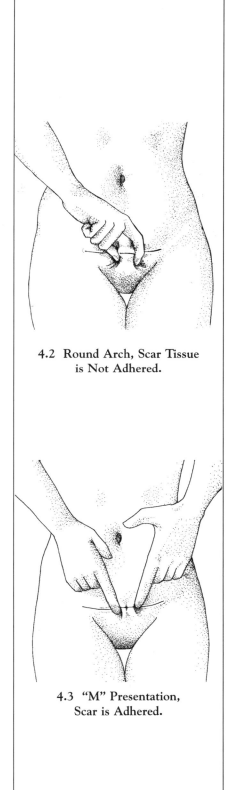

4.2 Round Arch, Scar Tissue is Not Adhered.

4.3 "M" Presentation, Scar is Adhered.

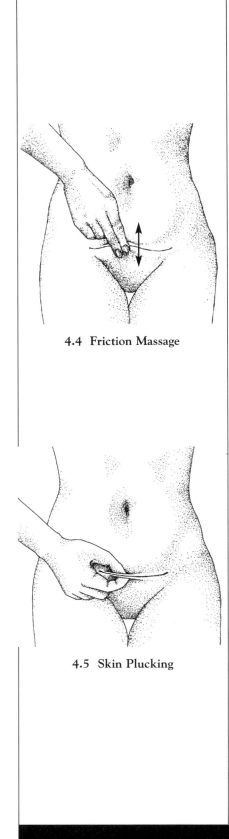

4.4 Friction Massage

4.5 Skin Plucking

If your cesarean incision goes up from the pelvic bone to the navel region, you will perform the massage techniques in a similar manner. Place your fingers perpendicular to your scar by placing your fingers sideways, instead of up and down.

4) **Friction Massage:** Place two fingers on the left side of your scar. Your fingers should be perpendicular to the scar. Gently pull the scar up toward your head, and push it down toward your feet in a rhythmic manner (see illustration 4.4). Hold 1/2 second or less n each direction. Avoid sliding your fingers across the skin. Your fingers should MOVE WITH THE SCAR. USE VERY LIGHT PRESSURE, APPROX. 2 - 3 OUNCES. Continue friction massage up to 2 minutes. Slowly raise your fingers off the scar. Repeat friction massage in the middle and right side of your scar.*

To perform friction massage on an episiotomy scar: WASH YOUR HANDS. Place your middle finger on the external episiotomy incision. Gently push the scar tissue side to side in a rhythmic manner. Hold 1/2 second or less in each direction. Avoid sliding your fingers across the skin. Your fingers should MOVE WITH THE SCAR. USE VERY LIGHT PRESSURE, APPROXIMATELY 2 - 3 OUNCES (about what you feel when you scratch your head). Continue friction massage up to 2 minutes. Repeat friction massage up and down the length of the incision.

*Please note that this type of massage is more prone to cause inflammation in the scar tissue. If you do notice that you have irritated your scar or surrounding tissue, discontinue or decrease the amount of time spent on this technique.

5) **Skin Plucking:** Lightly grasp one end of the scar between your thumb and index finger. Lift scar away from body, separating it from the underlying tissue (see illustration 4.5). Gently move your fingers side to side for 30 seconds. Move your fingers to the center of the scar, repeat technique, and then to opposite end of the scar, and repeat.

6) **Trigger Point Massage:** Locate a tender area and/or an area with a

small lump in the scar tissue or surrounding area. Place the tip of your thumb or middle finger on the bump. Lightly press down into the lump (see illustration 4.6). Hold 30 – 60 seconds. Slowly raise your thumb/finger. Please note, the fingers are moved to the side in the illustration, so that you can have a better view of the perineum. When performing trigger point massage on yourself, you may place your fingers on the perineum.

7) **Scar Tissue Taping:** A very new approach to reducing scar tissue without massaging the area is by placing kinesiotape, a very stretchy type of tape, onto the scar. Kinesiotape gently pulls the scar, separating it from underlying tissue (see illustration 4.7). Cut a piece of kinesiotape the length of your scar. Peel off the white backing. Gently stretch the tape until you feel a light resistance. Place stretched tape over the scar and adhere it to the scar/skin.

If you have a very sensitive scar, this is a nice way of gently breaking up adhesion without touching the area. This helps prepare you for other massage techniques. Scar taping is also wonderful because you may apply the tape and leave it on for 24 to 48 hours, or until it falls off. This tape applies a gentle pressure all the time, so it is working for you even while you work or sleep. To order a roll of kinesiotape, call (800) 523-0912.

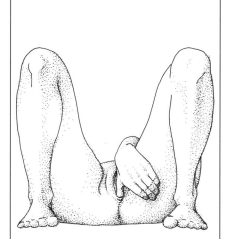

4.6 **Trigger Point Massage**

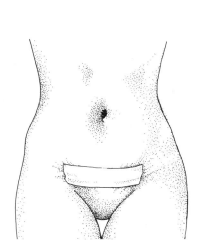

4.7 **Scar Tissue Taping**

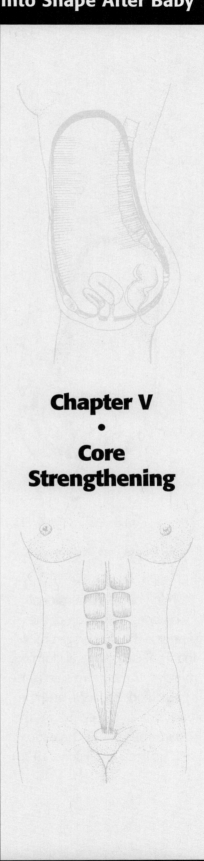

Chapter V
•
Core Strengthening

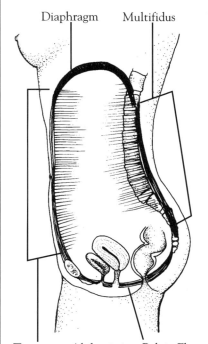

Diaphragm   Multifidus

Transverse Abdominis   Pelvic Floor

5.1 Core Stability Muscles

Think of a 3 dimensional cylinder, at the top of the cylinder is the diaphragm muscle, the front side is the abdominal muscles, the bottom side is the pelvic floor muscles, and the back side of the cylinder is the back muscles (Richardson, Jull, Hodges, and Hides, 1998).

Introduction to Core Strengthening

The exercises illustrated in this chapter will focus on the working relationship of the abdominal, back, diaphragm, and pelvic floor muscles. It is very important to learn how to use and properly strengthen these "core" muscles before progressing with an exercise program. To better understand the important role the abdominal, back, diaphragm, and pelvic floor muscles play in providing support and stability to your pelvis, spine, and abdomen, it is easiest to begin by identifying where all of these muscles are located.

Think of a 3 dimensional cylinder, at the top of the cylinder is the diaphragm muscle, the front side is the abdominal muscles, the bottom side is the pelvic floor muscles, and the back side of the cylinder is the back muscles (Richardson, Jull, Hodges, and Hides, 1998.) (see illustration 5.1).

The dome-shaped diaphragm muscle is the largest and primary breathing muscle. It separates the lungs from the abdominal cavity. When you breathe in, or inhale, the diaphragm muscle contracts and moves down, compressing the abdominal contents and increasing (intra-abdominal) pressure on your bladder, bowel, and pelvic floor muscles.

This is why women with weak pelvic floor muscles may leak urine when coughing, sneezing, jumping, etc. When you inhale, the diaphragm muscle pushes down, increasing pressure on pelvic floor muscles. If the muscles are weak, and cannot contract up against pressure, urine leaks out.

When exhaling, or breathing out, the diaphragm muscle returns to its dome shape causing a decrease in intra-abdominal pressure. It is easiest to contract pelvic floor muscles when there is less resistance or pressure. Pelvic floor muscles, therefore, must first be strengthened after or during exhaling, when the intra-abdominal pressure has decreased. When pelvic floor muscles become stronger, they can then be strengthened against intra-abdominal pressure, as while inhaling.

The transverse abdominis and multifidus muscles, part of the abdominal and back family muscles respectively, have been identified as being key muscles in stabilizing the spine (Richardson, Jull, Hodges, Hides,

1998). The transverse abdominis and multifidus muscles represent the abdominal and back muscles identified in illustration 5.1.

When the transverse abdominis muscle contracts, the abdomen moves toward the spine. This muscle acts as a corset to the abdominal contents, and assists with the stabilization of the spine. The contraction of the multifidus muscle is less discernable, however, it may be felt on both sides of the spine in the lower back region. This muscle keeps the spine in proper alignment, prevents excessive movement in the spine, and of course works with the transverse abdominis muscle in stabilizing the spine.

The transverse abdominis muscle has been shown to assist in the contraction of the multifidus muscle and vice versa (Richardson and Jull, 1995). In other words, if you are having a difficult time feeling and contracting the multifidus muscles as on page 125, try tightening your transverse abdominis muscle as on pages 123 and 124 strengthen the contraction of the multifidus muscle.

The pelvic floor muscles make up the base of the cylinder. Some of the pelvic floor muscles contract up and in, as with a Kegel exercise, or relax for voiding of urine and stool. As mentioned previously, the pelvic floor muscles must be able to work with or against the intra-abdominal pressure changes caused by the diaphragm muscle.

Interestingly enough, researchers have found a working relationship between the pelvic floor and the abdominal muscles, specifically the transverse abdominis muscles. It is speculated that the pelvic floor muscles work in unison with the multifidus (back) muscle as well. (Richardson, et. al 1998., Sapsford, et. al.1998, and Wilder 1993).

As you can see, the diaphragm, transverse abdominis, multifidus, and pelvic floor muscles all work together very closely. *Bounce Back Into Shape After Baby* focuses on strengthening your core (abdominal, back, diaphragm, and pelvic floor) muscles first because core muscle strength is necessary for proper posture, lifting and holding your baby, and performing any type of exercise. As basic exercises are mastered in this chapter, you may progress on to more dynamic exercises on the ball.

When the transverse abdominis muscle contracts, the abdomen moves toward the spine.

•

Interestingly enough, researchers have found a working relationship between the pelvic floor and the abdominal muscles, specifically the transverse abdominis muscles. It is speculated that the pelvic floor muscles work in unison with the multifidus (back) muscle as well. (Richardson, et. al 1998., Sapsford, et. al.1998, and Wilder 1993).

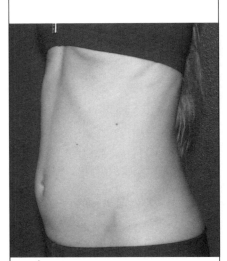

5.2 Relaxed Transverse Abdominis Muscle

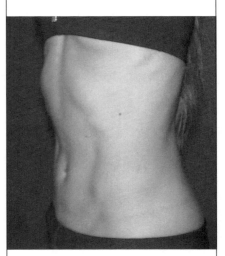

5.3 Contracted Transverse Abdominis Muscle

The remainder of this chapter includes helpful information on Weak Abdominal Muscles and Diastasis Recti, Back Pain, Diaphragmatic Breathing, Pelvic Floor Strengthening and Kegel Exercises. At the end of this chapter is a meticulously designed exercise program designed to address the abdomen, back, diaphragm, and pelvic floor muscles.

Weak Abdominal Muscles

Is your abdomen weak? Does it pooch out? Have you tried doing hundreds of sit-ups and you can't seem to get rid of your pooch, or worse – it becomes bigger? If so, you will definitely benefit from this chapter.

The majority of women, and men for that matter, can benefit from strengthening their abdominal muscles more effectively. Situps strengthen the most superficial layer of abdominal muscles. If you perform a situp when your deepest abdominal muscle layer, the transverse abdominis muscle, is weak, it is unable to act as a corset and function as a stabilizer to the abdomen.

Consequently, when performing a situp, the transverse abdominis muscle will cause the abdomen to bulge out and prevent the rectus abdominis muscle from tightening in an optimal position. When the transverse abdominis muscle becomes stronger, or is tightened while doing a situp, it is able to function as a corset and prevent the abdomen from bulging. Illustration 5.2 depicts the abdomen when the transverse abdominis muscle is relaxed, and illustration 5.3 depicts the transverse abdominis muscle when it is contracted. Notice how the back is less arched after the transverse abdominis muscle is tightened.

The secret to a successful abdominal strengthening program, and ridding yourself of an "abdominal pooch", is to strengthen the muscles from the inner to the outermost layers. The four different abdominal muscles, from inner to outermost layers, are the transverse abdominis, internal oblique, external oblique, and rectus abdominis muscles. Photographs were taken of each of these aforementioned muscles in a standing position.

- Transverse Abdominis - Innermost layer. Works in synergy (together) with the pelvic floor muscles. Assists with stabilizing, or controlling movement of the abdomen/spine before trunk, arms, or legs are moved. The waist narrows and the lower abdomen draws inward when the transverse abdominis muscle contracts, similar to the action of a corset (see illustration 5.4). To feel the transverse abdominis muscles, place your fingers just inside your hipbones. Contract the transverse abdominis as instructed on pages 123 or 124. You should feel the muscle tighten beneath your fingers. If your abdomen pooches out or bulges, try again, you are contracting the muscle incorrectly.

- Internal and External Obliques – Middle layers. These muscles work together to assist with rotation, side bending, and breathing, such as with Knee Rolls, page 141, Tummy Trimmin' Trunk Curl, page 152, and Diaphragmatic Breathing, page 45. The external oblique muscle assists with bowel movements by helping recruit rectal support for bowel emptying. The internal oblique is difficult to feel because it is located beneath the external oblique. To feel the external oblique muscle, place your hands on your hips. Contract the external oblique as instructed on page 126. You should feel your waist widen, pushing out into your hands (see illustration 5.5).

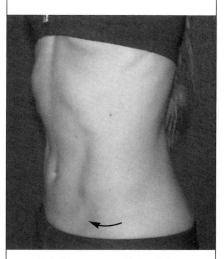

5.4 Transverse Abdominis –
Innermost Layer

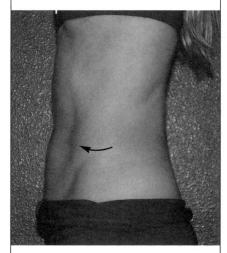

5.5 Internal and External
Obliques – Middle Layers

• Rectus Abdominis – Outermost layer. Flexes the trunk, as with a situp. This muscle may separate down the middle during pregnancy and cause a diastasis recti, see page 38. To feel your rectus abdominis muscle, lie on your back with knees bent. Place your hands in the middle of your abdomen. Lift your head off the floor. You should feel your abdomen tighten underneath your fingers (see illustration 5.6).

All of these aforementioned muscles become stretched and weakened during pregnancy. Therefore, it becomes paramount to learn how to contract each of these muscles independently of each other and strengthen them appropriately. Once you are able to strengthen your abdominal muscles properly, you will be on your way to developing a sleek, strong, and stabile abdomen.

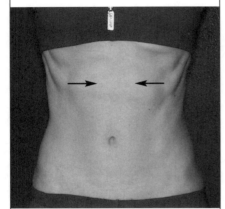

5.6 Rectus Abdominis –
Outermost Layer.

Once you are able to
strengthen your abdominal
muscles properly, you will be
on your way to developing
a sleek, strong, and
stabile abdomen.

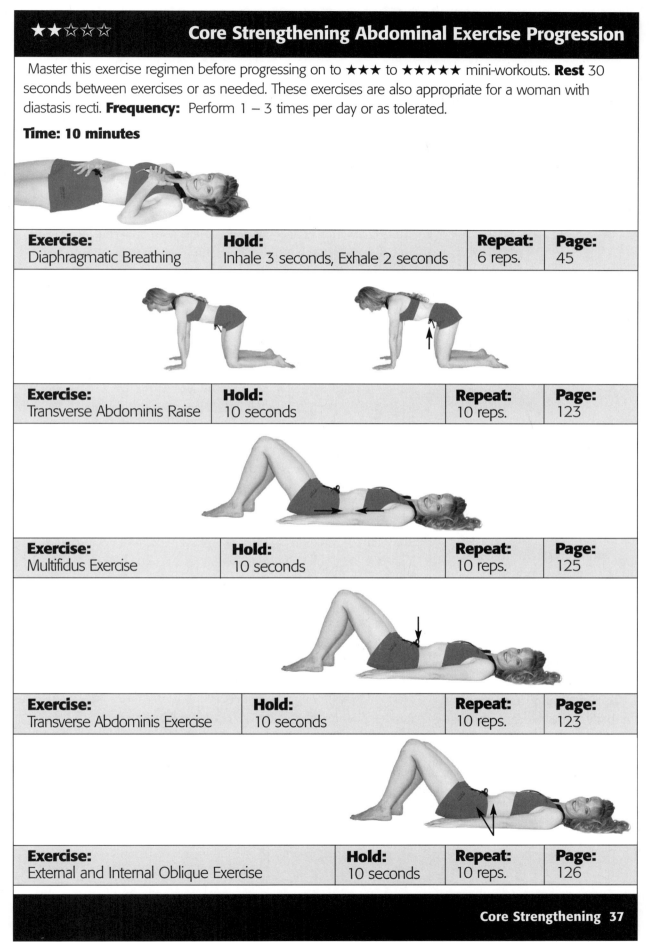

Master this exercise regimen before progressing on to ★★★ to ★★★★★ mini-workouts. **Rest** 30 seconds between exercises or as needed. These exercises are also appropriate for a woman with diastasis recti. **Frequency:** Perform 1 – 3 times per day or as tolerated.

Time: 10 minutes

Exercise:	Hold:	Repeat:	Page:
Diaphragmatic Breathing	Inhale 3 seconds, Exhale 2 seconds	6 reps.	45

Exercise:	Hold:	Repeat:	Page:
Transverse Abdominis Raise	10 seconds	10 reps.	123

Exercise:	Hold:	Repeat:	Page:
Multifidus Exercise	10 seconds	10 reps.	125

Exercise:	Hold:	Repeat:	Page:
Transverse Abdominis Exercise	10 seconds	10 reps.	123

Exercise:	Hold:	Repeat:	Page:
External and Internal Oblique Exercise	10 seconds	10 reps.	126

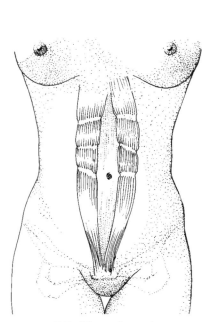

5.7 Diastasis recti

Two out of three women may experience a separation of the rectus abdominis muscle, the long muscle located in the middle of the abdomen, during their pregnancy

.

Since diastasis recti can predispose you to weak abdominal and trunk muscles, inability to do exercises properly, poor posture, and low-back pain, you will want to assess whether you have it or not.

Diastasis Recti

Two out of three women may experience a separation of the rectus abdominis muscle, the long muscle located in the middle of the abdomen, during their pregnancy (Boissonnault and Blaschak, 1988)(see illustration 5.7). This separation is called diastasis recti. The combination of abdominal weakness, hormonal changes, weight gain, and abdominal wall stretch exerted by your growing baby, can cause muscle separation along the centerline of the abdomen.

Diastasis recti most commonly occurs at the level of your umbilicus, or belly button. However, it may occur above or below the umbilicus or in a combination of these locations (Boissonault and Blaschak, 1988). The mid-line muscle separation usually happens during the second or third trimester of pregnancy, and may or may not resolve itself after the birth of your baby (Boissonault and Blaschak, 1988). You may not even be aware that you have a separation of the muscles. Several signs of a diastasis recti are: low-back pain, a small or large vertical bulge in the middle of your abdomen with standing and a gap or bulge in the same location when doing a situp.

Since diastasis recti can predispose you to weak abdominal and trunk muscles, inability to do exercises properly, poor posture, and low-back pain, you will want to assess whether you have it or not. To assess whether you have a separation of your abdominal muscles, please follow directions in the Diastasis Recti Self-Test on the next page.

If you or a healthcare professional has determined you have a diastasis recti, then you will need to perform exercises specifically designed to address it. Experts report that it may take from 1 to 4+ weeks for a muscle separation to resolve (Noble, 1998 and Gilleard and Brown, 1996). Gilleard and Brown further state that the ability of the abdominal muscles to stabilize the pelvis against resistance continues to be a problem 8 weeks after giving birth. Hence, they state, abdominal exercises should be chosen with care.

Follow the Diastasis Recti Exercise Progression as outlined on page 40 until your separation width of the rectus abdominis muscle is within one inch or no more than two fingers wide.

Diastasis Recti Self-Test

Target Area:
Rectus abdominis muscle, the long muscle located in the middle of the abdomen. (see illustration 5.8)

Benefits:
To determine if you have a vertical separation of the rectus abdominis muscle. Once a diastasis recti has been corrected, you will improve your posture, decrease your disposition to low-back pain, and enhance your aptitude to perform more difficult exercises correctly.

Avoid:
Avoid any strenuous activity or exercise until the diastasis recti is corrected to only two fingers width.

Instruction:
Lie on your back with your knees bent. Place four fingers of your left hand above belly button, and right hand below (see photograph 5.9). Raise your head and shoulders off floor. Is there a vertical separation of the rectus abdominis muscle, causing a gap of the muscles, and/or a bulge to appear? If so, where does the separation occur: above or below the umbilicus, or in a combination of these locations?

Now place four fingers, pointing toward floor, in the area of separation. Raise your head and shoulders off floor, reaching left hand out toward knee (see photograph 5.10). How many fingers can you place in the gap, one – two – three – four? Placing one to two fingers in the gap is normal. If you can place more than two fingers in the gap, you have a diastasis recti.

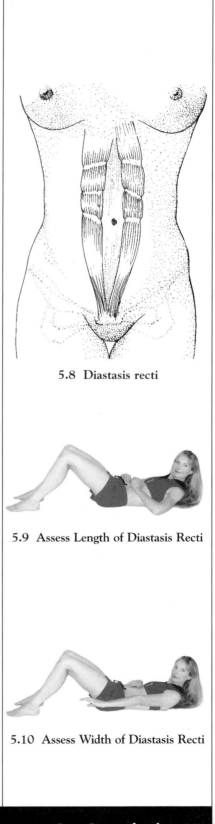

5.8 Diastasis recti

5.9 Assess Length of Diastasis Recti

5.10 Assess Width of Diastasis Recti

The following exercise progression is appropriate for a woman with diastasis recti. Progress to exercise number 5, neck curl, when you are able to do a neck curl without having a bulge, or diastasis recti. This exercise program is designed without a rest break between exercises.

Time: 4 minutes

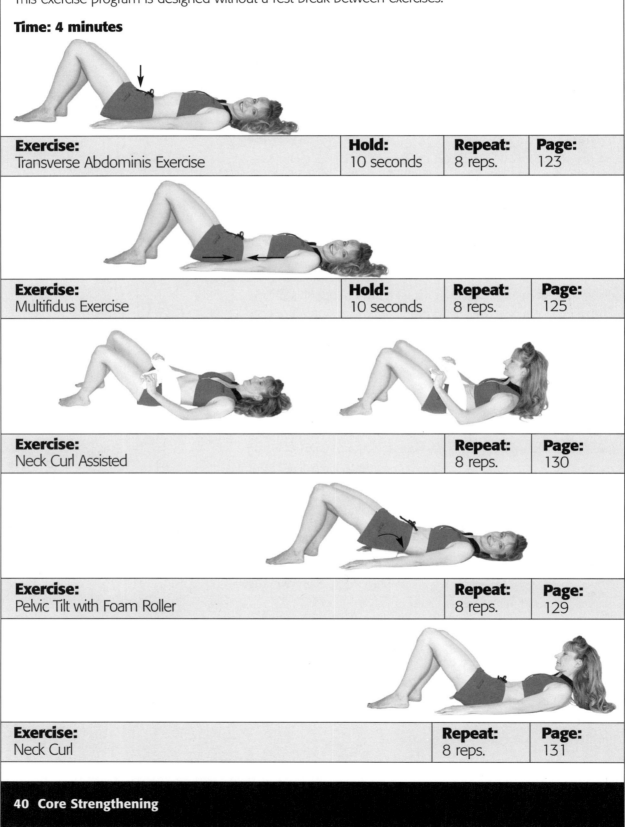

Exercise: Transverse Abdominis Exercise	Hold: 10 seconds	Repeat: 8 reps.	Page: 123

Exercise: Multifidus Exercise	Hold: 10 seconds	Repeat: 8 reps.	Page: 125

Exercise: Neck Curl Assisted		Repeat: 8 reps.	Page: 130

Exercise: Pelvic Tilt with Foam Roller		Repeat: 8 reps.	Page: 129

Exercise: Neck Curl		Repeat: 8 reps.	Page: 131

Back Pain

As many as sixty-seven percent of women have been reported to experience lower back pain after delivery (Ostgaard and Andersson, 1992). The majority of women's back pain resolved within the first 6 months after delivery, except women who experienced back pain in previous pregnancies. Of these women an astounding eighty-two percent continued to have back pain 18 months after childbirth (Ostgaard and Anderson, 1991).

Women appear to be at a higher risk for back pain if they are young, had back pain before or during their pregnancy, performed physically heavy work, or had more than one pregnancy (Berg, et. al., 1998, and Ostgard, and Anderson, 1991 and 1992).

Good posture, strong abdominal muscles, correct lifting habits (especially of your baby), and proper exercise techniques can prevent, reduce, or eliminate lower back pain. Please refer to chapters V, VII, and VIII for further information.

Hides, et. al., 1994, have found that the level of back pain correlates with wasting of the multifidus muscle, a very deep back muscle, at the same location as the pain. In other words, you are more likely to have weakness of the multifidus muscle at the location of your pain. Richardson, et. al., 1998, have found that back pain is reduced or eliminated with retraining or strengthening of the multifidus muscle.

Learn how to tighten the multifidus muscle first, as described on page 125, and follow the Lower Back Exercise Progression on page 42. Once you become proficient with these exercises, progress to ball exercises as illustrated in the strengthening chapter.

All of the lifting techniques and exercises request that you maintain a "neutral spine." To achieve a neutral spine, the lumbar spine (lower back) is not arched, nor is it rounded. A neutral spine is in between, providing the ability to strengthen muscles in an optimal position, avoid injury, and improve functional and athletic performance.

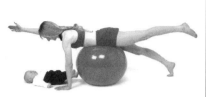

Back and Neck Strengthener, page 147.

As many as sixty-seven percent of women have been reported to experience lower back pain after delivery (Ostgaard and Andersson, 1992).

•

To achieve a neutral spine, the lumbar spine (lower back) is not arched, nor is it rounded. A neutral spine is in between, providing the ability to strengthen muscles in an optimal position, avoid injury, and improve functional and athletic performance.

Core Strengthening Lower Back Exercise Progression ★☆☆☆☆

Master this exercise regimen before progressing on to ★★★ to ★★★★★ mini-workouts. **Rest** 30 seconds between exercises or as needed. The following exercises are also appropriate for a woman with diastasis recti. **Frequency:** Perform 1 - 3 times per day or as tolerated.

Time: 10 minutes

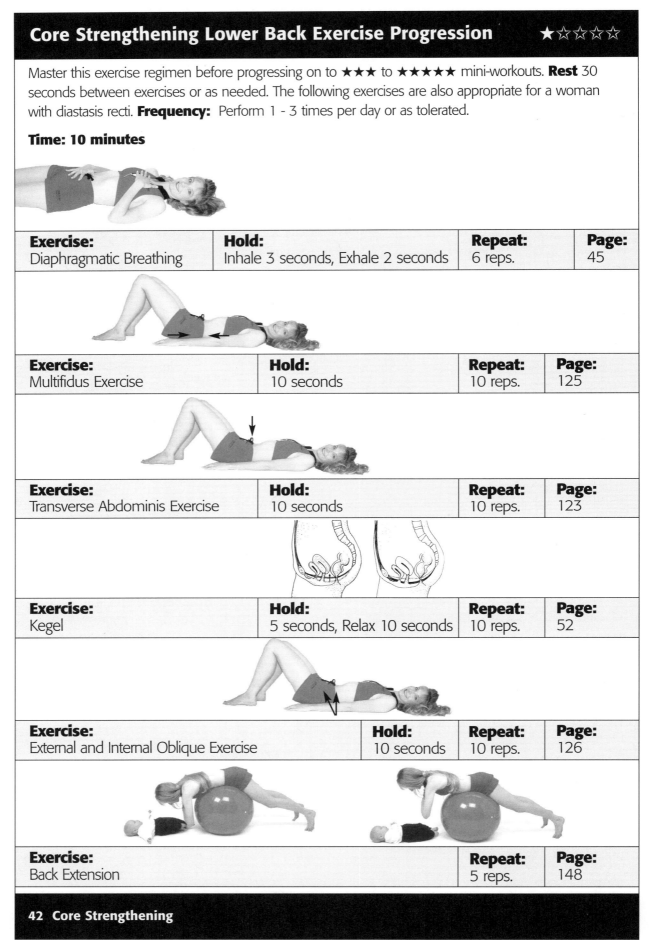

Exercise: Diaphragmatic Breathing	Hold: Inhale 3 seconds, Exhale 2 seconds	Repeat: 6 reps.	Page: 45

Exercise: Multifidus Exercise	Hold: 10 seconds	Repeat: 10 reps.	Page: 125

Exercise: Transverse Abdominis Exercise	Hold: 10 seconds	Repeat: 10 reps.	Page: 123

Exercise: Kegel	Hold: 5 seconds, Relax 10 seconds	Repeat: 10 reps.	Page: 52

Exercise: External and Internal Oblique Exercise	Hold: 10 seconds	Repeat: 10 reps.	Page: 126

Exercise: Back Extension		Repeat: 5 reps.	Page: 148

Diaphragmatic Breathing

Pregnant women require 10 to 20% more oxygen during their pregnancy, which necessitates a 40% increase in the amount of air that is inhaled and exhaled with each breath (ACOG, 1994 and Lindblom, 1995). This occurs, according to Dr. Laurie Lindbolm, by "breathing more deeply rather than more frequently." (Lindbolm, 1995). As the pregnancy progresses, the diaphragm muscle ascends with the increasing size of the baby, making it more difficult for diaphragmatic breathing to occur.

Diaphragmatic breathing, also known as belly breathing, is the correct form of breathing. Chest and shoulder breathing are very common methods of breathing during pregnancy and the postpartum period, despite the fact they are incorrect. The uterus presses up onto the diaphragm, making it more difficult to breathe. When it becomes difficult to breathe, instead of continuing with belly breathing, the body may compensate and start chest or shoulder breathing. Once your body has accommodated to chest or shoulder breathing, even after childbirth and the body has resumed a pre-pregnancy state, you may continue with this incorrect breathing pattern.

The average person breathes in and out 23,040 times per day! Imagine the tension that can develop in the chest or shoulder region when you are breathing incorrectly. Diaphragmatic breathing helps reduce muscular tension, promotes relaxation, and restores the working relationship between the pelvic floor, back, and abdominal muscles.

It is easiest to assess your breathing pattern in a quiet environment while comfortably positioned on your back. Loosen clothing, belts, or remove any other item that restricts the abdomen or causes irritation. A rolled towel or foam roller placed underneath the knees may further relax your body.

Pregnant women require 10 to 20% more oxygen during their pregnancy, which necessitates a 40% increase in the amount of air that is inhaled and exhaled with each breath (ACOG, 1994 and Lindblom, 1995).

•

The average person breathes in and out 23,040 times per day!

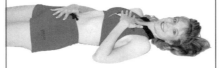

5.11 **Diaphragmatic Breathing**

Janet Hulme, P.T., recommends diaphragmatic breathing be performed for 30 - 60 seconds every hour throughout the day to help retrain the muscles (Creager, 1996, and Hulme, 1997)

•

Dr. Mark Schwartz, M.D., recommends repeating diaphragmatic breathing exercises "during the day as part of brief relaxations" and "any time you feel physically or emotionally tense" (Schwartz, 1987).

To determine which type of breathing pattern you use, gently rest one hand on your abdomen and one on your chest (see illustration 5.11). Where do you feel movement? If you feel your abdomen rising into your hand, you are most likely a diaphragmatic breather. If you do not feel any movement in your abdomen and lower ribs, you will need to re-train your breathing muscles.

Follow directions on the next page for diaphragmatic breathing. Once you can breathe diaphragmatically while lying on your back, progress to sitting and standing positions. Janet Hulme, P.T., recommends diaphragmatic breathing be performed for 30 - 60 seconds every hour throughout the day to help retrain the muscles (Creager, 1996, and Hulme, 1997). Dr. Mark Schwartz, M.D., recommends repeating diaphragmatic breathing exercises "during the day as part of brief relaxations" and "any time you feel physically or emotionally tense" (Schwartz, 1987).

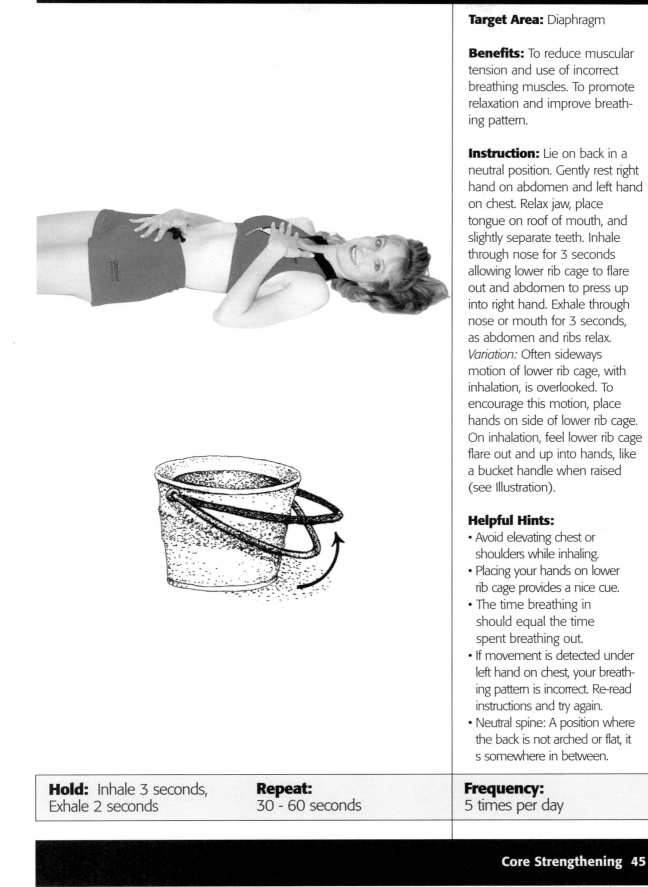

Target Area: Diaphragm

Benefits: To reduce muscular tension and use of incorrect breathing muscles. To promote relaxation and improve breathing pattern.

Instruction: Lie on back in a neutral position. Gently rest right hand on abdomen and left hand on chest. Relax jaw, place tongue on roof of mouth, and slightly separate teeth. Inhale through nose for 3 seconds allowing lower rib cage to flare out and abdomen to press up into right hand. Exhale through nose or mouth for 3 seconds, as abdomen and ribs relax. *Variation:* Often sideways motion of lower rib cage, with inhalation, is overlooked. To encourage this motion, place hands on side of lower rib cage. On inhalation, feel lower rib cage flare out and up into hands, like a bucket handle when raised (see Illustration).

Helpful Hints:
• Avoid elevating chest or shoulders while inhaling.
• Placing your hands on lower rib cage provides a nice cue.
• The time breathing in should equal the time spent breathing out.
• If movement is detected under left hand on chest, your breathing pattern is incorrect. Re-read instructions and try again.
• Neutral spine: A position where the back is not arched or flat, it s somewhere in between.

Hold: Inhale 3 seconds, Exhale 2 seconds

Repeat: 30 - 60 seconds

Frequency: 5 times per day

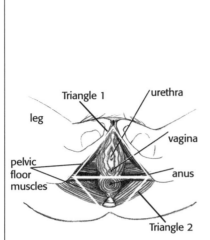

5.12 Pelvic Floor Muscles

The Agency for Health Care Policy and Research, 1994, reports that 87% of people who perform pelvic floor exercises significantly reduce or eliminate incontinence.

Pelvic Floor Strengthening and Kegel Exercises

Kegel exercises, developed by Dr. Arnold Kegel in the 1940s, are often recommended to strengthen the pelvic floor muscles. Strong pelvic floor muscles are imperative for support of pelvic organs, sexual sensation, and sphincteric control for continence of bowel and bladder. The Agency for Health Care Policy and Research, 1994, reports that 87% of people who perform pelvic floor exercises significantly reduce or eliminate incontinence.

Two types of muscle fibers make up the pelvic floor: fast and slow twitch fibers. This is significant because the fast and slow twitch muscle fibers enable you to perform different types of activities, and therefore must be strengthened in a distinct manner.

Fast twitch muscle fibers make up approximately 35% of the pelvic floor muscles, and are responsible for quick muscle contractions. Fast twitch muscle fibers are predominantly found in the triangle "1" location (see illustration 5.12) (Hulme, 1997). Fast twitch muscle contractions are rapid and explosive, yet short in duration, similar to a sprinter running a 100 meter dash. The Quick Flick exercise as discussed on page 56 is an example of a fast twitch muscle contraction. Perfecting this exercise will enable you to sneeze, cough, or jump without leaking urine.

Slow twitch muscle fibers comprise approximately 65% of the pelvic floor muscles, account for slow muscle contractions, and are primarily located in triangle "2" (see illustration 5.12) (Hulme, 1997). Slow twitch muscle contractions are required for endurance activities, such as standing throughout the day, or running a marathon. The Kegel exercise as shown on page 52 is an example of a slow twitch muscle contraction. Improving your 'hold' time for this exercise will make it possible for you to support your pelvic floor organs, maintain good posture, or sit/stand throughout the day without leaking urine. In addition, strengthening slow twitch muscle fibers will enhance your sexual sensation and ability to orgasm by allowing your pelvic floor muscles to squeeze the penis, please refer to the Sexersqueeze exercise on page 55.

Women often have difficulty coordinating the appropriate muscles to perform pelvic floor strengthening exercises. One of the most common mistakes women make when performing a Kegel exercise is to push the pelvic floor muscles down, instead of pulling them up and in (Bump, et. al., 1991). For this reason, it is important to perform the Start-Stop Tinkle Test, vaginal self-examination and/or perineum test, prior to initiating your pelvic floor strengthening program.

The Start-Stop Tinkle Test, page 50, has been included to help you identify your ability to start and stop your urine flow. This test will also help improve your awareness of which muscles you will need to use to tighten and relax pelvic floor muscles. This test is only a test and not an exercise. It is only to be completed ONE TIME PER MONTH to prevent disruption of the urinary tract reflex.

You may assess your pelvic floor muscles with a vaginal self-examination. Make sure you have thoroughly washed your hands before proceeding. Insert two fingers, or your thumb into the middle of your vagina. Perform a Kegel exercise, as instructed on page 52. You should feel your pelvic floor muscles lightly squeeze your finger. Now place your finger on each side of the vaginal walls and perform a Kegel. Do you feel that one side tightens more than another side? Right-handed women typically have stronger pelvic floor muscle contractions on the right side (Noble, 1995).

If you are uncomfortable with placing your finger in your vagina, you may try the perineum test. You will also assess your pelvic floor muscle contractions with the perineum test by placing your fingers on the perineum (the space between the vaginal and rectal opening). Once you have placed your fingers on the perineum, contract your pelvic floor muscles as instructed with the Kegel exercise, page 52. Do you feel the muscles move away from your fingers? If you feel the muscles bulge out and into your fingers you will need to consult with your obstetrician, obstetric physical therapist, and/or other health care professional, for further instructions on how to perform a Kegel exercise appropriately.

One of the most common mistakes women make when performing a Kegel exercise is to push the pelvic floor muscles down, instead of pulling them up and in (Bump, et. al., 1991).

•

Right-handed women typically have stronger pelvic floor muscle contractions on the right side (Noble, 1995).

Both the vaginal self-examination and perineum test can assist you in determining how many repetitions of each of the pelvic floor strengthening exercises you should perform. Perform a Kegel exercise and HOLD as long as you can. How long could you hold before your muscles fatigue? When fatigued, the vaginal walls will pull away from your fingers during the vaginal exam, or relax back down into your fingers on the perineum test. Perform the Quick Flick exercise and determine how many times you can perform the exercise before you fatigue.

Record this information, and it will help you determine how long you should hold and repeat the pelvic floor exercises. If you are performing a Quick Flick exercise and you are able to perform 6 repetitions before fatigue, and on the seventh repetition you begin to squeeze your buttocks and thighs, and clench your jaw, then it is time to stop. FATIGUE CAUSES MUSCLE SUBSTITUTION. Now you know to perform 6 repetitions the first set. Rest. Try and repeat 6 repetitions a second time.

You should gradually increase the HOLD time and/or repetitions of each exercise, if it is appropriate for the exercise, as your strength and endurance improve. Keep in mind it is not important how many repetitions of each exercise you do; it is important to perform the exercise properly without substitution of inappropriate muscles. Remember the phrase, Quality Not Quantity, when performing your pelvic floor exercises.

Many physical therapists recommend daily Kegel and pelvic muscle contractions, since pelvic floor muscles are used everyday during posture activities. However, if you find your pelvic floor muscles become overly fatigued from daily workouts, try performing these exercises every other day. Or perform different pelvic floor exercises each day. After you become proficient at doing these exercises, you may perform them every other day.

> Both the vaginal self-examination and perineum test can assist you in determining how many repetitions of each of the pelvic floor strengthening exercises you should perform.
>
> •
>
> You should gradually increase the HOLD time and/or repetitions of each exercise, if it is appropriate for the exercise, as your strength and endurance improve.
>
> •
>
> Many physical therapists recommend daily Kegel and pelvic muscle contractions, since pelvic floor muscles are used everyday during posture activities. However, if you find your pelvic floor muscles become overly fatigued from daily workouts, try performing these exercises every other day.

Your pelvic floor muscles are very important. Keeping them strong and healthy can prevent problems with your bowel and bladder later in life, especially throughout the hormonal changes of your menstrual cycle and menopause. Strong pelvic floor muscles can prevent and eliminate stress incontinence, support your pelvic organs, improve your sexual sensation and ability to orgasm during intercourse. Continuing the pelvic floor strengthening exercises as instructed in this book, pages 51 – 58, throughout your lifetime is good preventative self-care.

"Pelvic floor muscles need to work at the right time and to be strong enough for the demands each woman places upon them. Core stability demands slow twitch activity, that can be maintained over a period of time. Once this is functioning, then strengthening work is added to the muscle, usually by a stronger hold sustained for 5 – 6 seconds.

It is now known that an independent transverse abdominis muscle contraction recruits a slow twitch pelvic floor contraction. Once more abdominal muscles (the obliques) are recruited isometrically, the strength of the pelvic floor contraction increases. If one is attempting to retrain the pelvic floor muscles, the order should be slow twitch holds first, and once these are achieved (say able to hold easily for 15 seconds), then strengthening should be added. This can be done by either conscious strong pelvic floor contractions (pages 51–57), or by increasing strength of isometric abdominal contractions (pages 123, 124 and 126). Instructions to avoid contraction of the abdominal muscle will not get the best pelvic floor strength. It seems that pelvic floor rehabilitation is not complete until the abdominal wall is also rehabilitated.

The women with the strongest pelvic floor have strong abdominal isometric holds (as on pages, 123,124 and 126), all without doing specific pelvic floor exercises. They may also have strong dynamic abdominal activity too. I now rehabilitate the pelvic floor by using this programme."

– personal communication, Ruth Sapsford, 2001.

Target Areas:
Pelvic floor and sphincter muscles.

Benefits:
To determine your ability to start and stop urine flow.
To improve awareness of and ability to tighten and relax pelvic floor muscles.

Instruction:
Sit on toilet and start urinating. Stop the flow of urine midstream by contracting/tightening your pelvic floor muscles. Start the flow of urine, and stop once again.

Repeat:
Start and stop the urine flow 3 times. This test is only to be completed ONE TIME PER MONTH to prevent disruption of the urinary tract reflex.

Hints:
• Avoid performing this test your first trip to the bathroom in the morning.
• If you are vertically challenged and find your feet dangling while you sit on the toilet, place a phone book under your feet for support. This position will make you more relaxed while performing test.
• If you have a urinary tract infection (UTI), discontinue exercise. When the UTI has resolved, you may once again perform this test.

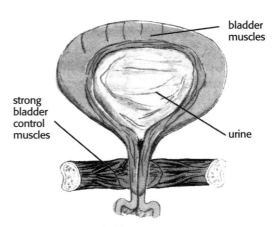

Strong Bladder Control Muscles

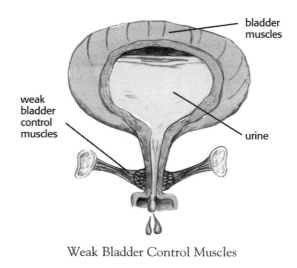

Weak Bladder Control Muscles

Hold:	**Repeat:**	**Frequency:**
3 seconds	3 times	One time per month

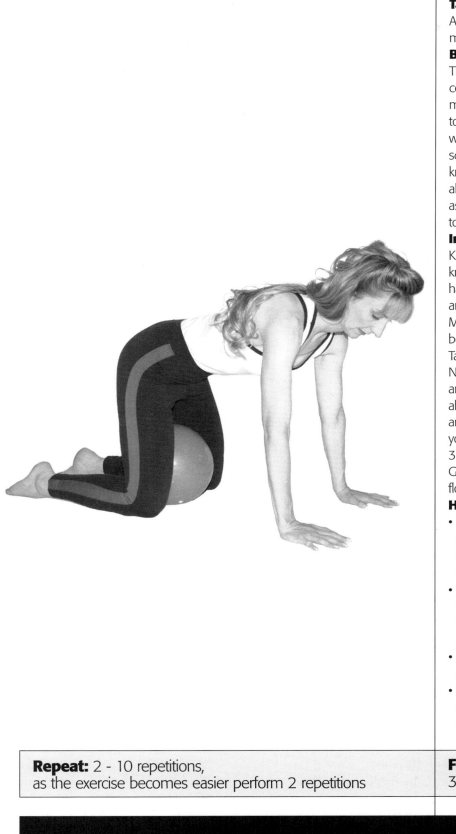

Target Areas:
Abdomen and pelvic floor muscles.

Benefits:
This exercise helps the abdominal corset (transverse abdominis muscle) and pelvic floor muscles to work in unison. If you have weak pelvic floor muscles, lightly squeezing the ball with your knees and contracting your abdominal corset muscles will assist the pelvic floor muscles to tighten.

Instruction:
Kneel. Place 20 cm. ball between knees. Lean forward and place hands on floor. Align shoulders and hands, and hips and knees. Maintain head alignment with body, and a neutral spine position. Take a relaxed breath in and out. Now without breathing in, slowly and gently draw the lower abdomen in towards the spine and squeeze the ball between your knees. Hold this position for 3 - 20 seconds, breathe lightly. Gradually relax abdomen, pelvic floor and legs.

Helpful Hints:
• This is a very gentle exercise. If you pull lower abdomen up too far, internal oblique muscles will be recruited.
• When you can hold this exercise for 20 seconds, progress to the Transverse Abdominis raise on page 124.
• Avoid movement of the trunk or pelvis while performing exercise.
• Neutral spine: A position where the back is not arched or flat, it is somewhere in between.

Repeat: 2 - 10 repetitions, as the exercise becomes easier perform 2 repetitions

Frequency: 3 times per day

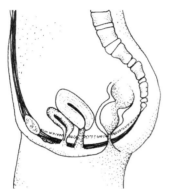

Pelvic Floor At Rest

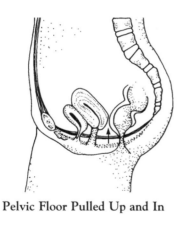

Pelvic Floor Pulled Up and In

Target Areas:
Pelvic floor and sphincter muscles.

Benefits:
To support the pelvic floor region and improve pelvic floor muscle strength and endurance, as with maintaining good posture, standing/sitting throughout the day. To gain awareness of how to use and coordinate pelvic floor muscles.

Instruction:
Lie down on back with knees bent and feet shoulder-width apart. Take a relaxed breath in and out. Now without breathing in, slowly draw the pelvic floor muscles up and in as if you are attempting to stop urine flow. Inhale. Hold this position for 3 seconds. Gradually relax the pelvic floor muscles for 6 seconds. Repeat exercise as above, however, slowly draw the pelvic muscles up and in as if you are preventing gas from escaping. Hold this position for 3 seconds. Gradually relax the pelvic floor muscles. Relax for 6 seconds, and repeat exercise.

Helpful Hints:
• Your relaxation period should be twice as long as your hold time, until you approach a 10 second hold. That is, if you can hold your Kegel for 5 seconds, you should relax for 10 seconds or if you can hold your Kegel for 10 seconds, your relax time should be 10 seconds.
• Exercise Progression: Once you have mastered this exercise, progress to doing the exercise sitting, standing, or squatting.
• Avoid movement or contraction of the abdominal, buttock, and/or inner thigh muscles while performing exercise.
• If you have difficulty contracting pelvic floor muscles, try this exercise lying on your side lying (equivalent to ★). You may also place your finger inside the vagina, and try to squeeze your finger, or try the Sexersqueeze exercise.

Hold: 3 Seconds, increase to 15 seconds gradually

Repeat: 3 – 10 reps.

Frequency: 3 times a day or whenever the phone rings

Target Areas:
Pelvic floor and sphincter muscles.

Benefits:
To gain awareness of how to use and coordinate pelvic floor muscles, and disassociate pelvic floor muscles from diaphragm. To support pelvic floor region, and improve pelvic floor muscle strength and endurance, as with maintaining good posture standing/sitting throughout the day.

Instruction:
Lie down on back with knees bent and feet shoulder-width apart. Take a relaxed breath in and slowly draw pelvic floor muscles up and in for 5 seconds, as if you are attempting to stop urine flow. Gradually relax pelvic floor muscles during exhalation for 5 seconds. Repeat exercise as above, however, slowly draw the pelvic muscles up and in as if you are preventing gas from escaping. Hold this position for 3 seconds. Gradually relax the pelvic floor muscles. Relax for 5 seconds, and repeat exercise.

Helpful Hints:
• Your relaxation period should be twice as long as your hold time, until you approach a 10 second hold. That is, if you can hold your Kegel for 5 seconds, you should relax for 10 seconds or if you can hold your Kegel for 10 seconds, your relax time should be 10 seconds.
• Exercise Progression: Once you have mastered this exercise, progress to doing the exercise sitting, standing, or squatting.
• Avoid movement or contraction of the abdominal, buttock, and/or inner thigh muscles while performing exercise.
• If you have difficulty contracting pelvic floor muscles, try this exercise lying on your side (equivalent to ★★). You may also place your finger inside the vagina and try to squeeze your finger, or try the Sexersqueeze exercise.

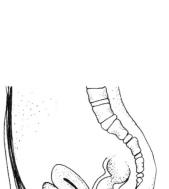

Pelvic Floor At Rest

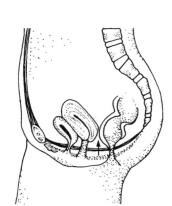

Pelvic Floor Pulled Up and In

Hold: 5 seconds breathing in, 5 seconds breathing out	**Repeat:** 3 to 10 reps	**Frequency:** 3 times a day

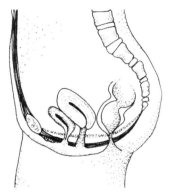

Pelvic Floor At Rest

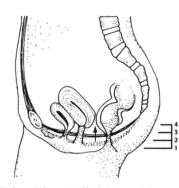

Pelvic Floor Pulled Up and In

Target Areas:
Pelvic floor and sphincter muscles.

Benefits:
An advanced exercise to improve slow twitch pelvic floor muscle strength and endurance. To gain awareness of how to use and coordinate pelvic floor muscles.

Instruction:
Lie down on back with knees bent and feet shoulder width apart. Inhale. Take a relaxed breath in and out. Now without breathing in slowly draw the "elevator" or pelvic floor muscles up and in. Follow directions as above. Visualize raising an elevator to the first floor. Hold this position for 2 seconds. Gently breathe in and out while holding the pelvic floor muscles tight. Raise the elevator to the 2nd floor, 3rd floor, and 4th floor. Hold for 2 seconds on each floor. Gradually relax the pelvic floor muscles as if descending one floor at a time. Hold relaxation period for 10 seconds and repeat exercise.

Helpful Hints:
• Exercise Progression: Once you have mastered this exercise, progress to doing the exercise sitting, standing, or squatting.
• Avoid movement or contraction of the abdominal, buttock, and/or inner thigh muscles while performing exercise.

Hold:
2 seconds on each floor
Relax: 8 seconds
Frequency: 3 times a day

Repeat:
1 - 5 repetitions. If you have difficulty raising the elevator to the fourth floor, gradually increase the number of floors the elevator can ascend and descend.

Target Area:
Pelvic floor muscles.

Benefits:
To improve pelvic floor muscle strength and endurance.
To gain awareness of how to use and coordinate your pelvic floor
muscles. To improve your sensation during sex by strengthening
pelvic floor muscles that 'squeeze' the penis.

Instruction:
Choose a sexual position of your preference. After penile penetration,
take a relaxed breath in and out. Now without breathing in, squeeze the
penis with your vaginal muscles. Gently breath in and out while holding
the pelvic floor muscles tight. Hold this position for 3 seconds. Gradually
relax the pelvic floor muscles. Rest for 10 seconds. Repeat.

Variation:
Follow directions as above, however, perform the "Quick Flick exercise"
during penile penetration. Repeat 3 – 10 quick flicks in rapid succession.
Relax. Repeat until fatigue, and/or partner reports less squeezing action.

Helpful Hints:
• Progress length of time you hold Kegel contraction from 3 seconds to
  15 seconds. Once you are able to maintain a pelvic floor contraction
  for 15 seconds, repeat the exercise up to 10 times.
• Avoid movement or contraction of the abdominal, buttock, and/or
  inner thigh muscles while performing exercise.

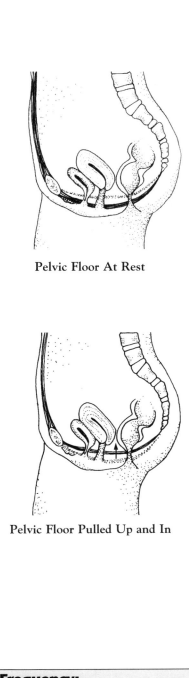

Pelvic Floor At Rest

Pelvic Floor Pulled Up and In

Hold: 3 seconds, rest 6 seconds, increase to 15 seconds gradually.	**Repeat:** Until fatigue, and/or partner reports less squeezing action.	**Frequency:** To be determined by user.

Quick Flick Kegel

★★☆☆☆

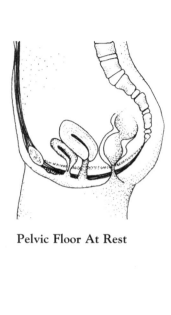

Pelvic Floor At Rest

Quick Flick Muscles Pulled Up and In

Target Areas:
Pelvic floor and sphincter muscles.

Benefits:
This exercise strengthens (fast twitch) pelvic floor muscles and helps prevent urine leaking while coughing, sneezing, jumping, lifting etc.

Instruction: Lie down on back with knees bent and feet shoulder width apart. Take a relaxed breath in and out. Now without breathing in, quickly flick pelvic floor muscles up and in. Focus on completely relaxing muscles. Always anticipate your cough or sneeze! To prevent urine from leaking, quick flick before coughing or sneezing.

Helpful Hints:
• Avoid movement or contraction of the abdominal, buttock, and/or inner thigh muscles while performing exercise.
• Exercise Progression: Once you have mastered this exercise, progress to doing the exercise sitting, standing, or squatting.
• If you have difficulty contracting pelvic floor muscles, try this exercise lying on your side (equivalent to ★). You may also place two fingers inside your vagina and try to squeeze your fingers.

Hold:
1 second, Relax: Completely

Repeat:
2 - 10 reps.

Frequency: 3 times per day or just before you sneeze

Target Area:
Pelvic floor muscles.

Benefits:
Strengthens pelvic floor muscles. This exercise may help prevent 'urine leaking' while coughing, sneezing, jumping, lifting, etc., and assist with defecating.

Instruction:
Lie down on back with knees bent and feet shoulder-width apart. Take a relaxed breath in and out. Now without breathing in, raise anus up and move tailbone side to side. Visualize moving tailbone to right knee. Relax. Repeat. Draw anus up and move anus to left knee. Hold. Relax.

Helpful Hints:
• Avoid movement or contraction of the abdominal, buttock, and/or inner thigh muscles while performing exercise.
• If you are having difficulty performing this exercise, place fingers on each side of tailbone and perform an External Oblique exercise. You should feel the same muscles used for "tail wagging."
• *Exercise Progression:* Once you have mastered this exercise, progress to doing the exercise while sitting, standing, or squatting.

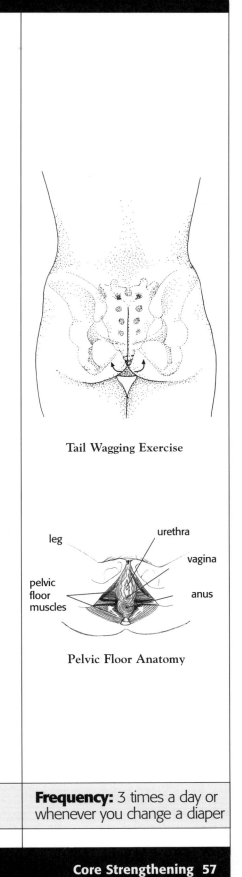

Tail Wagging Exercise

Pelvic Floor Anatomy

Hold: 1 second, Relax completely	**Repeat:** 2 – 10 times	**Frequency:** 3 times a day or whenever you change a diaper

Performing a pelvic floor exercise workout is more difficult than doing the exercises individually. Master individual exercises before performing this mini-workout. Perfect this exercise regimen before progressing on to ★★★ to ★★★★★ mini-workouts. **Rest** 60 seconds between exercises or as needed.
Frequency: Perform 1- 3 times per day or as tolerated.

Time: 10 minutes

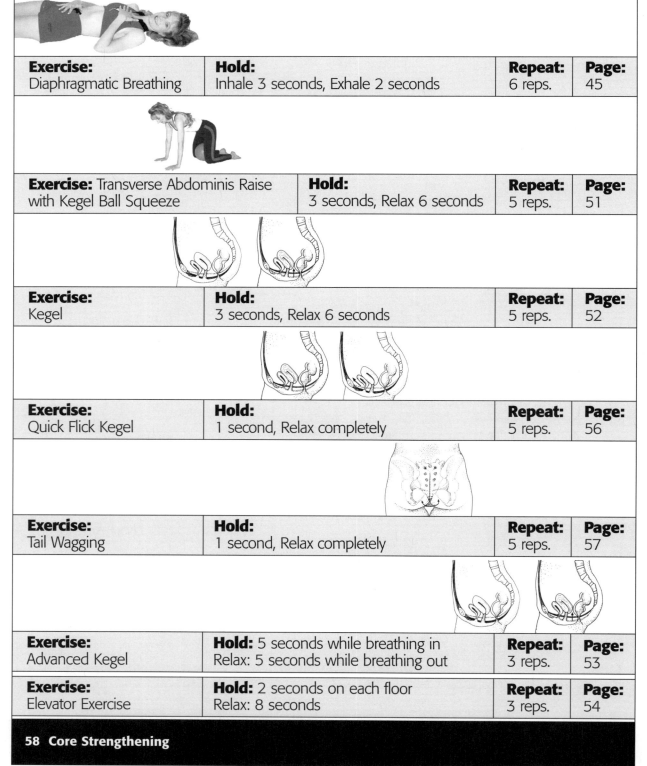

Exercise: Diaphragmatic Breathing	**Hold:** Inhale 3 seconds, Exhale 2 seconds	**Repeat:** 6 reps.	**Page:** 45
Exercise: Transverse Abdominis Raise with Kegel Ball Squeeze	**Hold:** 3 seconds, Relax 6 seconds	**Repeat:** 5 reps.	**Page:** 51
Exercise: Kegel	**Hold:** 3 seconds, Relax 6 seconds	**Repeat:** 5 reps.	**Page:** 52
Exercise: Quick Flick Kegel	**Hold:** 1 second, Relax completely	**Repeat:** 5 reps.	**Page:** 56
Exercise: Tail Wagging	**Hold:** 1 second, Relax completely	**Repeat:** 5 reps.	**Page:** 57
Exercise: Advanced Kegel	**Hold:** 5 seconds while breathing in Relax: 5 seconds while breathing out	**Repeat:** 3 reps.	**Page:** 53
Exercise: Elevator Exercise	**Hold:** 2 seconds on each floor Relax: 8 seconds	**Repeat:** 3 reps.	**Page:** 54

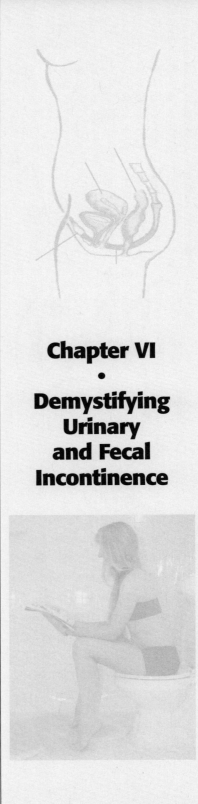

Chapter VI
•
Demystifying Urinary and Fecal Incontinence

Introduction to Incontinence

What does i-n-c-o-n-t-i-n-e-n-c-e really mean? Urinary incontinence simply means an involuntary loss or accidental leakage of urine. More than 15 million people in North America experience urinary incontinence (Wilkes, 1999). Studies have shown that as many as 52% of women experience urinary incontinence (Bo, 2000), and are more than twice as likely to experience incontinence than men (Wilkes, 1999). Morkved and Bo (1999) report the prevalence of urinary incontinence during pregnancy at 42%. Thirty-eight percent of these women continued to report urinary incontinence 8 weeks after delivery.

Fecal incontinence is the involuntary loss of gas or stool from the anus. MacArthur, et. al., (2001) studied the prevalence of fecal incontinence. They found that almost 10% of the women they interviewed reported fecal incontinence 3 months after childbirth.

Pregnancy, childbirth, and the structure of the female urinary tract are all contributing factors to urinary and fecal incontinence.

Pelvic floor muscles, located from the pubic bone to the tail bone, form a hammock-like sling that keep your uterus, bladder, and bowel supported (see illustration 6.1). Specialized sphincter muscles encircle the openings of the bladder and rectum and assist in controlling the openings to these organs (see illustration 6.2). The sphincter muscles act as a faucet – opening to allow urine and bowel movements to pass and closing when not needed. Strong pelvic floor muscles (see illustration 6.3) also assist in keeping the urethra, the tube that carries urine from your bladder down to an opening in front of the vagina, and rectum closed.

In order for urine and feces to be released, the urethral and anal sphincter muscles and surrounding pelvic floor muscles must relax voluntarily. The bladder should stay relaxed when it is full of urine. However, when you are ready to urinate, the bladder muscle should tighten and squeeze urine out. Feces are pushed out with the assistance of the abdominal (external and internal oblique) muscles and intra-abdominal pressure created by the abdominal and diaphragm muscles.

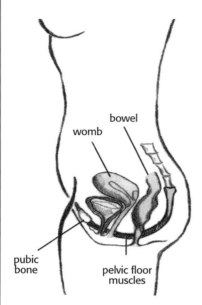

6.1 Lower Abdomen

More than 15 million people in America experience incontinence (Wilkes, 1999). Studies have shown that as many as 52% of women experience urinary incontinence (Bo, 2000), and are twice as likely to experience incontinence than men (Wilkes, 1999).

Your pelvic floor muscles should be strong and tight to hold up your bladder and rectum in their proper place. It is difficult for the pelvic floor muscles to do their job of supporting the pelvic contents and controlling urination and bowel movements when they are weak or stretched. Weakened pelvic floor muscles may allow the rectum, bladder, uterus, and/or urethra to shift down, out of their original place, causing incontinence.

Urinary Incontinence

The most common type of urinary incontinence during pregnancy or after delivering your baby is stress incontinence. Stress incontinence is the involuntary loss of small amounts of urine (from several drops to a dribble) following a sudden increase in intra-abdominal pressure, such as with sneezing, coughing, laughing, or physical activity. Weak sphincter or bladder control muscles may suddenly relax when you are sneezing. The weak sphincter muscles may be unable to squeeze the urethra completely closed and consequently allow urine to travel through the urethra – leaking urine.

Some stress incontinence is not unusual during pregnancy and after delivering your baby. There are many reasons why it is so common: weak pelvic floor muscles, fatigue, hormonal changes during pregnancy, and tissue stretch, stress, and tears during labor and delivery.

Stress incontinence is also more prevalent during the week before your period. It is not your imagination, lowered estrogen levels during this time or during menopause may lead to lower muscular pressure around the urethra, increasing chances of leakage.

Urge incontinence is defined as the involuntary loss of urine associated with a strong urge to urinate at unexpected times, such as when going from a sitting to a standing position, or arriving home and walking into your house, or as you sleep.

There are many types of urinary incontinence. The common types of urinary incontinence are summarized in the table below.

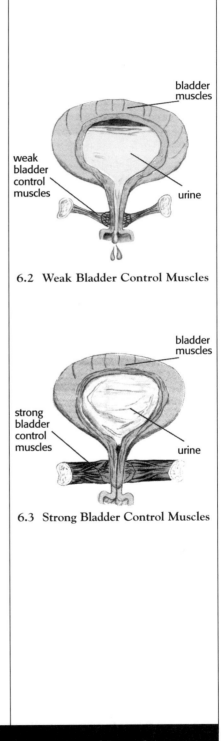

6.2 Weak Bladder Control Muscles

6.3 Strong Bladder Control Muscles

Common Types of Urinary Incontinence

Stress: Leakage of small amounts of urine during physical movement or activity, as with coughing, sneezing, jumping, and lifting. You may avoid exercise because you are afraid of "leaking".

Urge: Leakage of large amounts of urine at unexpected times, such as when you hear running water, going from sitting to standing, or while you sleep. You may go to the bathroom every two hours and may wet the bed at night.

Functional: Untimely urination because of physical disability, external obstacles, or problems with thinking or communicating that prevent you from reaching the toilet. This may be caused by multiple sclerosis, spinal cord injury, dementia, etc.

Overflow: Unexpected leakage of small amounts of urine because of a full bladder. You may dribble urine throughout the day, or feel the urge to urinate, but at times cannot.

Mixed: Combination of both stress and urge incontinence.

Transient: Temporary leakage of urine that occurs as a result of a medical condition that will improve or go away - as with yeast and/or urinary tract infections, mental impairment, stool impaction, and/or medication.

The Agency for Health Care Policy and Research, 1996, reports that 80% of urinary incontinence can be helped by non-invasive techniques. Strengthening the pelvic floor muscles with exercise usually eliminates pregnancy related stress incontinence within several months following delivery. Urge incontinence may take longer to resolve, and may require medical intervention. Please refer to the 15 Steps to Continence for additional treatment options.

Constipation and Fecal Incontinence

Constipation is prevalent in women who have recently had a baby. Constipation in the post-partum woman is most likely due to weak pelvic floor muscles. Strengthening pelvic floor muscles, increasing activity level, eating high fiber foods, and drinking plenty of water will usually resolve constipation problems.

Fecal incontinence is often caused by a severe tear of the perineum during childbirth. Women who receive midline episiotomies are 4.2 to 12 (younger women vs. older women) times more likely to experience a rupture of the anal sphincter than women who receive mediolateral incisions (Shiono, et. al., 1990). Women who deliver by forceps have almost twice the risk of developing fecal incontinence as compared with women who did not have a forceps delivery.

One of the most basic ways to prevent constipation and improve fecal incontinence is to learn proper toilet voiding techniques. Please refer to the Toilet Training Techniques on the next page for further details. Anyone can benefit from these techniques, especially women who have just given birth. Additional basic treatment techniques for fecal incontinence are listed in the 15 Steps to Continence. I encourage women who experience fecal incontinence to follow up with their healthcare professional for further treatment options.

Toilet Training Techniques

Adapted from *Women's Health: A Textbook for Physiotherapists,* Sapsford et. al., Physiotherapy Management of Pelvic Floor Dysfunction, pp. 397 – 399, 1998, by permission of the publisher Bailliere Tindall.

Target Areas:
External and internal obliques (side abdominal), transverse abdominis (side and front), rectus abdominis (front), diaphragm, pelvic floor, and anal sphincter muscles.

Benefits:
This toilet positioning technique improves the defecation pattern by widening the angle of the rectum and the opening of the anus, and assisting with relaxation of the outer anal sphincter muscle, and the pelvic floor muscles.

Instruction:
Sit on toilet with knees more than shoulder-width apart. Place feet on foot stool if knees are not above hips. Lean forward placing forearms on knees. Maintain a neutral spine position. <u>Allow your abdomen to bulge</u> by relaxing the rectus abdominis muscle. Raise heels up (see illustrations 6.3 and 6.4).

If you need to **Push** to empty the bowel, the following should occur as you push:
1. your waist widens sideways
2. abdomen bulges forward
3. back remains upright as depicted
4. pelvic floor muscles descend about 1 inch (2 – 3 cm.) and then hold firm
5. anal sphincter muscles relax
6. rectal emptying occurs
7. feel your body with your hands, try to distinguish each of these movements when they occur

Helpful Hints:
• Avoid straining and a rounded back position.
• Avoid dangling feet. Use a footstool. Orthopedic Physical Therapy (800-530-6878) sells a nice foam wedge that is perfect for foot placement.
• If the pelvic floor muscles seem to descend more than one inch (2 – 3 cm.) and emptying requires more effort, support the perineum with your hand during bowel movement.
• Neutral spine: A position where the back is not arched or flat, it is somewhere in between.

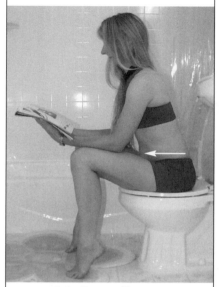

6.3 Correct Position

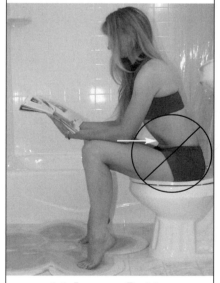

6.4 Incorrect Position

How are Urinary and Fecal Incontinence Treated?

Many basic treatment options are available for women who experience stress, urge, or fecal incontinence. Please refer to 15 Steps to Continence. I urge all women who have problems with incontinence, pelvic pain, and/or have difficulty performing the pelvic floor strengthening exercises recommended in this book to please consult your obstetrician, obstetric physical therapist, and/or other healthcare professional for further treatment options.

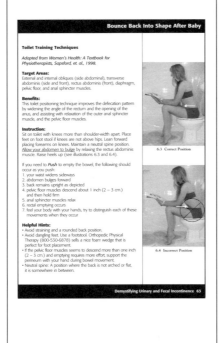

15 Steps to Continence

(SI = Stress Incontinence, UI = Urge Incontinence, and FI = Fecal Incontinence)

1. Perform pelvic floor exercises as recommended in *Bounce Back Into Shape After Baby*. SI, UI, FI

2. Empty your bladder and bowel before exercise or intercourse. SI, FI

3. Cross your legs or press your hand over your clitoris when you have the urge to urinate. UI

4. Avoid straining while trying to void urine or stool. Follow proper Toilet Training Techniques. UI, FI

5. Discuss a bladder training program with your healthcare professional. UI

6. Void urine every 3 – 4 hours. The average person voids 8 times per day. UI

7. Set an alarm to wake yourself up one time per night. UI

8. Insulate cold toilet seats by placing toilet paper or cushion on seat. When a cold surface touches your skin, it causes a reflexive action to tighten your muscles, not relax them. Consequently, urinating or defecating becomes more difficult. UI, FI

9. Monitor fluid intake. The average person should drink 8 glasses, 1.5 – 2 liters, per day. UI

10. Participate in a relaxation training program. SI, UI, FI

11. Eat plenty of fiber. FI

12. Avoid caffeine and alcohol. UI, FI

13. Monitor intake of medication. Some types of medication cause constipation and/or make the bladder more active. UI, FI

14. Discuss the option of receiving electrical stimulation and/or biofeedback treatments with your healthcare professional. Both of these treatment techniques have been shown to improve stress, urge, and fecal incontinence. SI, UI, FI

15. Talk to your healthcare professional to ascertain whether special medications, pessaries (A special device that is inserted into the vagina to support the bladder and prevent urine leakage), and/or surgery are options for you.

Chapter VII

•

Look Like You Have Lost 10 Pounds by Improving Your Posture

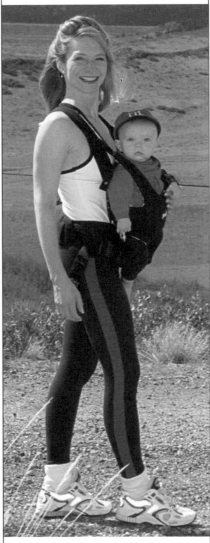

7.1 Stand Up Straight

Do You Still Look Like You Are Pregnant?

Rid yourself of at least 10 pounds by STANDING UP STRAIGHT (see illustration 7.1). This sounds so simple, but due to pregnancy and poor posture habits your body may not remember what it is like to 'stand and sit tall' with good alignment.

The rounded pregnant look is most often caused by a combination of weak muscles, weight gain, rounded shoulders, and a forward tilted pelvis. These changes, plus the dramatic shift in the center of gravity, contribute to the typical 'arched back, rounded shoulder' pregnancy stance.

How will this poor post-partum posture affect you? Muscles that were not intended to work full time may be constantly working as substitutes. The consequence of this may be low back pain, knee pain, wrist pain, and poor habitual posture.

The most habit forming post-partum posture happens as a result of an arched back. The key to correcting an arched back (or flat back for that matter) is to first learn where your "neutral spine" position is. What is a "neutral spine" position? To achieve a neutral spine, the lumbar spine (lower back) is not arched, nor is it rounded. A neutral spine is in-between, providing the ability to strengthen muscles in an optimal position, avoid injury, and improve functional and athletic performance.

I recommend you begin with a 3-Step Posture Check to improve your posture. Everyday, throughout the day, do posture checks to make sure you are exhibiting the posture that makes you feel best, and the posture you want other people to see. My 3-Step Posture Check consists of: 1) Raise Your Chest, 2) Roll Back Your Shoulders and, 3) Tighten Your Abdominal Muscles.

The key to good posture, and the 3-Step Posture Check is to be able to maintain proper posture through out the day. In order to attain and maintain proper posture throughout the day you will need to do a few exercises that correspond to the 3-Step Posture Check. If you do the 3-Step Posture Check without doing the exercises, you will probably have a difficult time maintaining your newly attained good posture.

Pregnancy, breast and bottle-feeding, lifting, and holding baby all require carrying additional weight in front of the body. These activities cause the shoulders to droop and the back to round. In order to be able to RAISE YOUR CHEST and maintain this position, you will first need to stretch your chest and arm muscles.

1. The Chest, Arm, and Finger Stretch helps you to RAISE YOUR CHEST and pull back your shoulders.

One of the weakest areas of a woman is in her mid-back region. Women who have weak mid-back muscles are likely to slouch or exhibit poor posture. In order to ROLL BACK YOUR SHOULDERS, you will need to strengthen your mid-back and shoulder muscles.

2. ROLL BACK YOUR SHOULDERS and maintain this position by strengthening your neck, mid-back, and shoulder muscles with the Shoulder Rowing exercise.

After giving birth many women arch their low back. This happens due to the abdominal muscles lengthening and weakening during pregnancy. Tightening and strengthening the abdominal muscles, in conjunction with strengthening the back and buttocks, will eliminate the sway back posture.

3. The Transverse Abdominis Raise exercise will strengthen and TIGHTEN ABDOMINAL MUSCLES.

Good posture exudes self-confidence, positive energy and makes you appear more fit and attractive. Follow the 3-Step Posture Check, and perform the Posture Perfect Exercise Program as instructed on the next page, and you will be on your way to attaining and maintaining good posture for life.

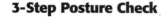
3-Step Posture Check

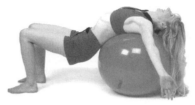
1. Chest, Arm, and Finger Stretch (Refer to page 107).

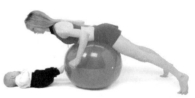
2. Shoulder Rowing (Refer to page 144).

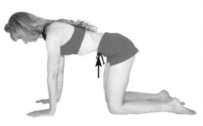
3. Transverse Abdominis Raise (Refer to page 124).

Posture Perfect Exercise Program ★★☆☆☆

The following exercise program is wonderful for a woman who exhibits the typical post-partum posture: rounded shoulders, chin and ribs down, and an arched back. This exercise program is designed without a rest break between exercises. **Frequency:** 1 – 2 times per day.

Time: 5 minutes

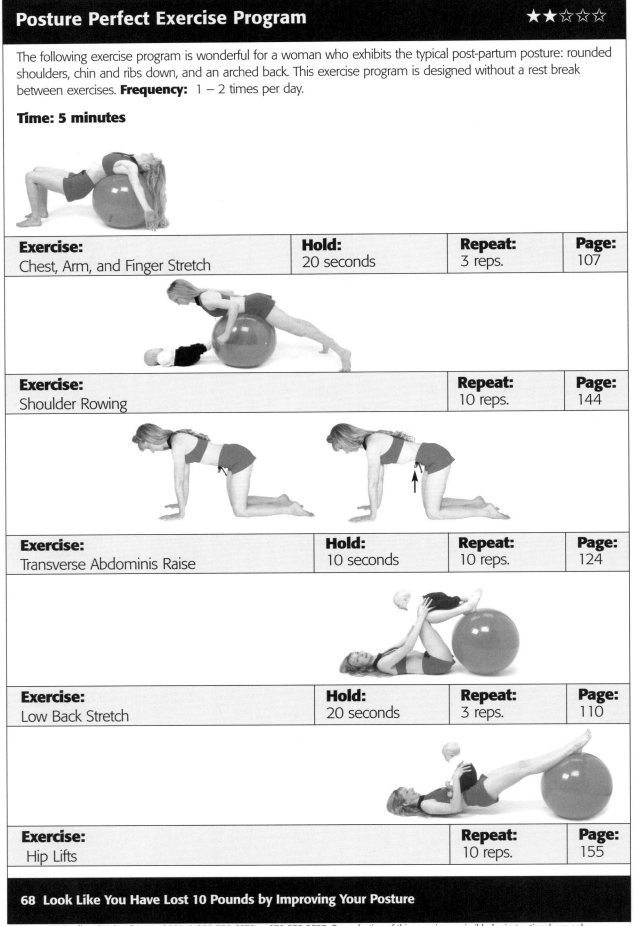

Exercise:	Hold:	Repeat:	Page:
Chest, Arm, and Finger Stretch	20 seconds	3 reps.	107

Exercise:		Repeat:	Page:
Shoulder Rowing		10 reps.	144

Exercise:	Hold:	Repeat:	Page:
Transverse Abdominis Raise	10 seconds	10 reps.	124

Exercise:	Hold:	Repeat:	Page:
Low Back Stretch	20 seconds	3 reps.	110

Exercise:		Repeat:	Page:
Hip Lifts		10 reps.	155

Chapter VIII
•
Proper Body Mechanics for Lifting and Holding Your Baby

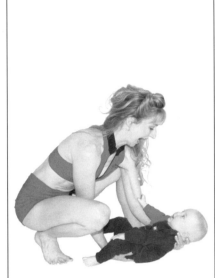

On an average day,
I lift a minimum of
771 pounds without
even using weights!
- Caroline Creager

•

More than 80% of the
population experiences
back pain at least
once in their lifetimes.

The Importance of Good Body Mechanics

How many times during the day do you lift your baby into and out of the crib, off the floor, or in and out of the car? I found that during an average 24-hour period, I placed my son in and out of the crib 15 times, placed him on and lifted him off the floor 10 times, placed him on and lifted him off the changing table 16 times, lifted him into and out of the car, with car seat, 6 times, and held him for approximately 2.5 hours (this includes feedings). Wow, lifting and carrying your baby throughout the day is a workout in itself.

On an average day, I lift a minimum of 771 pounds without even using weights! I arrived at this number by calculating the number of times I lifted my son on average in a 24-hour period, and multiplying this number by his weight (See chart below). The amazing thing is, this number does not even include lifting my 31 pound two year old.

More than 80% of the population experiences back pain at least once in their lifetimes. As you can see, post-partum women are at high risk for developing low back, upper back, neck, and pelvic floor pain. This is why it is absolutely essential to lift and carry your baby properly.

	My Son's Weight		Number of Lifts			
In/Out Crib -	15	x	15	=	225 pounds	(102 kilograms)
On/Off Floor -	15	x	10	=	150 pounds	(68 kilograms)
On/Off Changing Table -	15	x	16	=	240 pounds	(109 kilograms)
In/Out Car - (with car seat)	26	x	6	=	156 pounds	(71 kilograms)
TOTAL WEIGHT LIFTED:				**=**	**771 pounds**	**(351 kilograms)**

Take a few moments to think about how you hold your baby. Do you hold your baby in your arms in front of your body, or do you rest him/her on your hip? One of the most common practices for carrying a baby is depicted in illustration 8.1. Mom thrusts out her hip and rests the baby on her hipbone. Most right-handed women place their baby on their left hip. This position may cause low back, hip, or knee pain due to the thrusting and hiking of the hip, and rotational motion of the back.

Many times you will find the need to place your baby on your hip. If you do, just try not to thrust your hip out. Keep your hips aligned over your knees. The front hold and straddle hold are preferred holding positions.

How do you lift your baby off the floor or changing table? You will need to ask yourself all of these questions. The next few pages will give you an opportunity to learn more about alternate holding (carrying) and lifting positions and their benefits. You will also be able to identify recommended exercises from this book and how they help you better perform everyday activities with your baby.

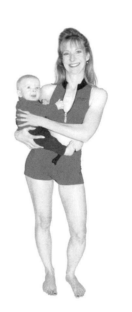

8.1 Improper Baby on Hip Position

Target Areas:
Arms, abdomen, and back.

Benefits:
This position more evenly distributes baby's weight throughout your body reducing stress on back, knees, and hips. Baby also benefits from this position. Baby improves his/her reflexes, neck, back, and leg strength by holding his body up against gravity.

Instruction:
Turn baby on his/her tummy. Place both forearms under baby. Clasp hands underneath baby to give yourself more leverage. Hold baby as close to body as possible. Keep shoulders back, and chest elevated. Tighten tummy by pulling belly button in towards spine. Baby is ready to see the world as an airplane.

Variation:
When baby is still small you may hold him over one forearm. This will allow you to work with the opposite hand. Remember to alternate placing baby on right and left forearms.

Helpful Hint:
Avoid arching back or rounding shoulders.

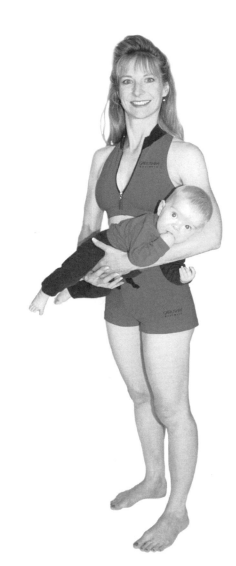

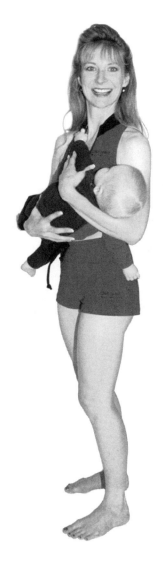

Target Areas:
Arms, abdomen, and back.

Benefits:
Your baby can see the expressions on your face more clearly and you are able to interact with your baby. Your baby can also hear your heart beat.

Instruction:
Place baby, tummy-up, in your arms. Hold baby as close to body as possible. Keep shoulders back, and chest elevated. Tighten tummy by pulling your belly button in towards spine. Alternate placing baby's head in left and right arm.

Helpful Hint:
Avoid arching back or rounding shoulders.

Target Areas:
Arms, abdomen, and back.

Benefits:
The Front-Facing and Straddle Hold Positions are ideal alternatives to placing baby on hip. These positions alleviate low back, hip, or knee pain by preventing your hip from hiking and your back from rotating.

Instruction:
Place baby in a front-facing position as depicted in Photo A, or a front-straddle position as depicted in Photo B. Hold baby as close to your body as possible. Keep shoulders back and chest elevated. Tighten tummy by pulling belly button in towards spine.

Helpful Hint:
Avoid arching back or rounding your shoulders.

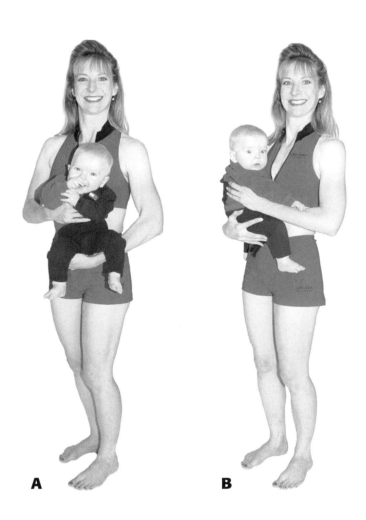

A

B

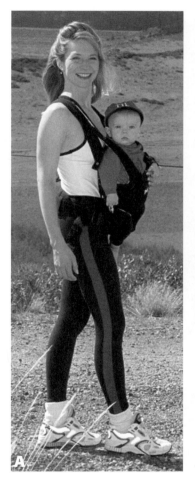
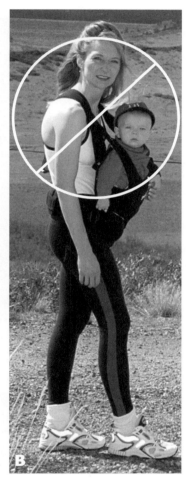

Target Areas:
Abdomen, chest, upper, middle, and lower back, and neck.

Benefits:
A front pack is an excellent way to carry baby around the house so you can have the use of your hands. A front pack is also a wonderful way of carrying your child so you can freely swing your arms while walking. The free-swinging arm motion helps strengthen abdominal muscles.

Instruction:
Place baby in a front pack. Lift baby and place front pack straps over shoulders. Secure waistband with latch, and tighten to comfort. Tighten front pack straps so baby is as close to your body as possible. Keep shoulders back, and chest elevated. Tighten tummy by pulling your belly button in towards spine. Walk with arms swinging freely.

Helpful Hints:
• If possible, have your partner hold baby while you wiggle into front pack straps.
• The front facing baby position is a more advanced position for baby, and is designed for a baby who has good head control (can lift head up and maintain position). When baby is first born, you will need to place baby in front pack, so his/her tummy touches yours.
• A front pack may be used until baby reaches about 14 pounds. At this time you will need to transition him/her to a back pack (only if your child has good head control), or a baby stroller.
• When you become fatigued, shoulders will start to droop. This will be your key to finish your walk.

Squat Lift

Target Areas:
Abdomen, back, neck, and pelvic floor.

Benefits:
The squat lift strengthens legs which guards against low back strain.

Instruction:
Stand with one foot in front of other. Bend knees. Place one hand under baby's head and opposite hand under buttocks region. Tighten abdominal muscles by pulling belly button towards spine. Exhale as you lift baby off floor, and bring baby to chest. Tighten leg muscles and stand up. Maintain good posture by keeping a neutral spine.

Helpful Hints:
- Avoid twisting your back.
- You should feel the squat lift in your legs, and not your back. If you feel discomfort in your back when lifting baby, you may need to strengthen your legs. Try the standing squat exercise on page 77.
- You may also roll baby onto his/her side or tummy, and lift baby from floor in this position.

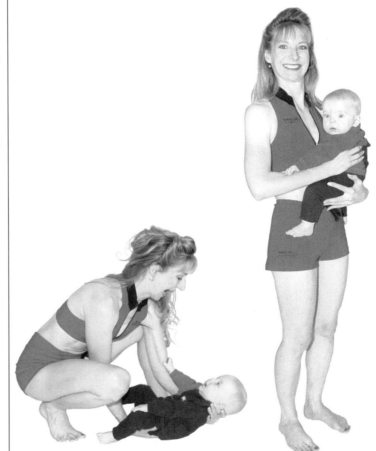

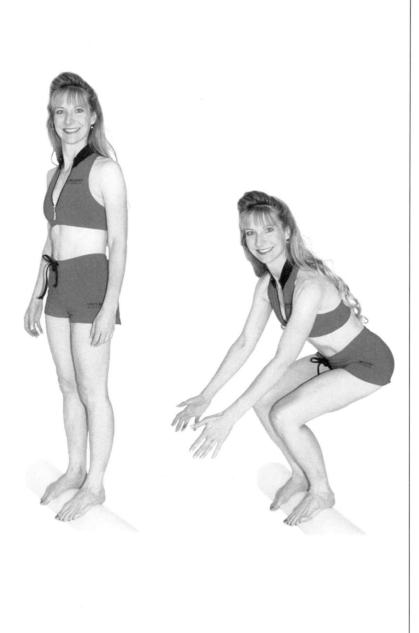

Target Areas:
Abdomen, back, neck, and pelvic floor.

Benefits:
One of the easiest ways to learn how to properly perform a standing squat is to stand on a foam roller and bend your knees. This exercise will improve balance and naturally help re-align your spine.

Instruction:
Stand with roller horizontal on floor in front of body. Place one foot at a time on roller. Stand on roller with feet shoulder-width apart. Tighten abdominal muscles by pulling belly button towards the spine. Exhale as you bend knees slightly and raise arms out in front of you, as if you were going to lift your baby. Return to standing position. Tighten your abdominal muscles by pulling belly button towards spine. Exhale, and perform a Quick Flick exercise as instructed on page 56.

Helpful Hints:
- NEVER perform this exercise holding baby.
- ALWAYS have someone spot you.
- Begin this exercise 6 weeks post-partum, when your ligaments are not as lax, or as directed by your physician.
- Begin with a 3 foot long half-roller with the flat surface up (equivalent to ★★★), and progress to a 3 foot long round roller as depicted (equivalent to ★★★★).

Hold: 5 seconds	**Repeat:** 3 – 12 times X 2 reps	**Frequency:** 2 times per day or before brushing your teeth

Target Areas:
Lower and upper back.

Purpose:
This lift strengthens legs, which helps guard against low back strain.

Instruction:
Lower crib rail. Stand as close to the crib as possible. Place one foot in front of other. Lean forward, bending knees and hips. Place one hand under baby's head and opposite hand under buttock region. Tighten abdominal muscles by pulling belly button towards spine. Exhale as you lift baby out of crib, and bring baby to chest. Tighten leg muscles and stand up. Maintain good posture by keeping a neutral spine.

Helpful Hints:
• Avoid twisting your back.
• You should feel the squat lift in your legs, and not your back. If you feel discomfort in your back when lifting your baby, you may need to strengthen your legs. Try the standing squat exercise on page 77.
• You may also roll baby onto his/her side or tummy, and lift baby from crib in this position.

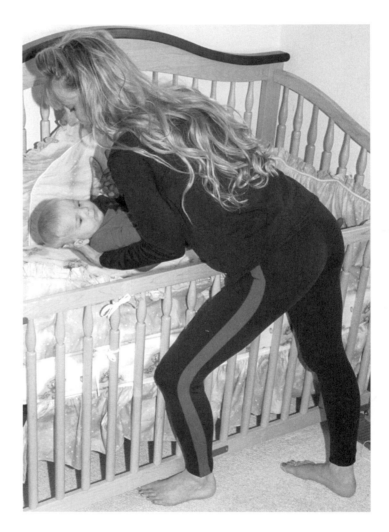

Target Areas:
Abdomen and back.

Benefits:
Car lifts are one of the most difficult lifts a new mother must perform. Advance planning on how you are going to lift your child in and out of the car is recommended. This car lift will minimize low back, abdominal, and pelvic floor strain.

Instruction:
To lift baby out of car, stand as close to vehicle as possible. If baby is positioned in far right seat, raise right foot and place it in the inside of the car. Lean body into car transferring weight onto right foot. Release baby carrier from base. In preparation for lifting baby out of base, place right hand on bottom of car seat, and left hand on carrier handle. Tighten abdominal muscles by pulling belly button towards spine. Exhale and lift child in carrier as close to body as possible. Transfer weight to back left foot, as you raise your right foot and place it on ground.

If baby is in middle car seat position, climb into car. Follow directions as above, however place left knee on car seat, and right foot on floor with knee bent. Keeping baby as close to body as possible, scoot backward to edge of car on knee. Place baby on car seat. Climb out of car. Tighten abdominal muscles by pulling belly button towards spine and perform a Kegel exercise. Exhale and lift child as close to body as possible.

Helpful Hints:
• Keep baby rear facing until she/he is 20 pounds.
• Remember, if you have just had a cesarean delivery, avoid lifting your child in and out of car.

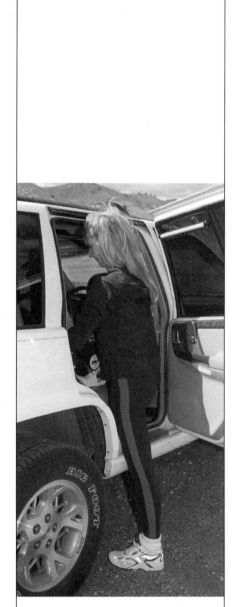

Proper Lifting and Holding Positions for Your Baby At a Glance

The following lifting and holding positions illustrate good body mechanics. By using good body mechanics throughout the day, you will strengthen your muscles in an optimal position, avoid injury, and improve functional performance.

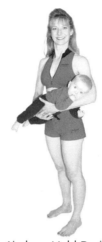

Airplane Hold Position

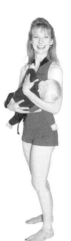

Breast-feeding Hold Position

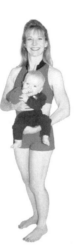

Front-facing Hold Position

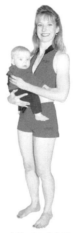

Straddle Hold Position

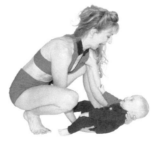

Squat Lift

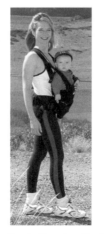

Front Pack Carrying Position

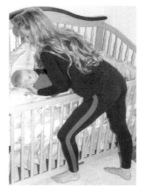

Crib or Changing Table Lift

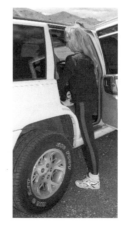

Car Lift

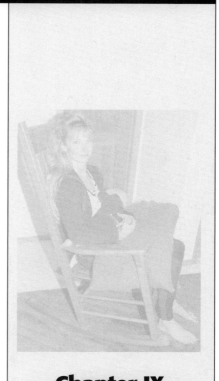

Chapter IX
•
Breast-feeding
and Exercise

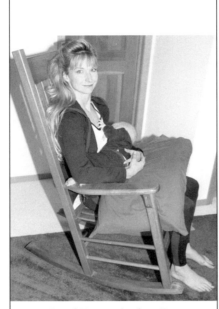

9.1 Good Breast-feeding Position

Breast-feeding exclusively for the first 3 months reduces the risk of obesity in children, decreases the number of ear infections, and likelihood of developing asthma, diarrhea, and other childhood illnesses (von Kreis, 1999).

•

"In our 15-year experience, less than two percent of women who exercise during pregnancy feed formula to their offspring."
–James F. Clapp III, M.D.

The Importance of Breast-feeding

The good news is that you can safely exercise if you are breast-feeding your baby. Moderate exercise does not decrease the quality of your breast milk or the supply available to your baby (Prentice, 1994). And don't worry about your baby not liking the taste of your breast milk after you have exercised, my babies never complained – sweat and all.

I have to admit that at first I was not sure whether or not breast-feeding was something I was really interested in doing, especially since I like to exercise. Since I read research studies stating that breast-feeding exclusively for the first 3 months reduces the risk of obesity in children, decreases the number of ear infections, and likelihood of developing asthma, diarrhea, and other childhood illnesses (von Kreis, 1999), I realized how important it is to breast-feed your baby. I decided to make the commitment, to myself, that I would breast-feed my first child for at least 6 months. I surprised myself and breast-fed him for one year. My second child is 3 months old and I'm still breast-feeding him.

I soon found out that breast-feeding was a wonderful bonding experience for both my babies and myself. I felt like I was providing both of my children with something no one else possibly could, mom's milk – the most easily digested nutrition source filled with immunity building properties, and lots of love.

It is a challenge to fit in a workout between breast-feeding sessions, however in the long run it is worth it for both you and your baby. Fifty-eight percent of women in the United States breast-feed their babies (United States Department of Health and Human Services, 1996). Interestingly enough, women who exercise are more likely to breast-feed than women who do not exercise. Dr. James Clapp III, a renowned researcher in the area of exercise and pregnancy, states that "in our 15-year experience, less than two percent of women who exercise during pregnancy feed formula to their offspring." (Clapp, 1998).

When breast-feeding your baby, assume a good posture by placing a pillow under the baby when she/he is small (see illustration 9.1).

The pillow brings the baby's mouth closer to your nipple, and allows you to relax more by keeping your shoulders back. As your baby grows, you will be able to eliminate the pillow and still keep good posture.

A few reasons not to exercise when you are breast-feeding include: breast infection/ abscess, breast pain, and substantial reduction in milk production. If you have breast pain, you may be experiencing a plugged milk duct, an infection, or an abscess. Increased circulation, as with exercise, may spread the infection. If you have any questions as to whether you may have an infection, please call a lactation specialist or your physician.

Breast discomfort is usually caused by engorgement of the breast tissue. Your breasts will feel heavier than normal and especially so when full of milk. Emptying your breasts before exercise will increase your comfort. I usually breast-feed my son before I exercise and if this is not an option I express milk with a breast pump. Remember to save and freeze the expressed milk for use in the future!

Sports Bras

For your own comfort, you will not want to bounce on the ball or schedule vigorous aerobic exercise when your breasts are full or engorged. The extra jostling can be uncomfortable, and may lead to stretching of the breast tissue.

You will want to invest in a good quality, supportive sports bra. The following tips will help you find the proper bra for you and your body:
- Find one that gives good support without tightly binding your breasts.
- Wide shoulder straps help distribute the weight of your breasts more evenly on your shoulders. This will help prevent neck, shoulder, and upper back pain.
- Select one that supports both breasts evenly without cutting into them. If there is an indentation or red mark on your shoulder, the bra is too tight.

A few reasons not to exercise when you are breast-feeding include: breast infection/ abscess, breast pain, and substantial reduction in milk production.

•

Emptying your breasts before exercise will increase your comfort.

•

Wide shoulder straps help distribute the weight of your breasts more evenly on your shoulders. This will help prevent neck, shoulder, and upper back pain.

H$_2$O

The body needs extra water when exercising and even more if you are producing breast milk. The demands of breast-feeding plus the demands of exercise absolutely require you to drink lots of water!

Fatigue and "dry mouth" are symptoms of dehydration. To prevent dehydration, drink at least eight ounces (one cup) of water after exercise, and continue to drink water at regular intervals throughout the day. A lactating woman who exercises should drink a minimum of 16 8 ounce glasses of water a day; that's 4 quarts or 8+ pounds of water a day. Water constitutes approximately 57% of your total body weight (Guyton, 1987).

Keep in mind that beverages that contain caffeine or alcohol may tend to cause dehydration as well as disrupt sleep. (Although when you are sleep deprived like myself, as soon as my head touches the pillow, I fall fast asleep).

Temporary Calcium Loss

Breast milk is high in calcium. Some of that calcium may come from your bones. This can result in transient bone loss. This is a temporary situation and resolves itself when your baby is weaned. We do know that weight-bearing exercise is good for your bones. Weight bearing applies muscle stress to the bone and strengthens the bone where the muscle is attached.

You should not have to take extra calcium supplements if you exercise while breast-feeding. Several studies have shown that calcium 'bio markers' (used to measure calcium in the bones) were not affected by calcium supplements. After breast-feeding was discontinued, the bone calcium levels return to homeostasis, with or without calcium supplementation. (Kalkwarf, et. al., 1999).

> To prevent dehydration, drink at least eight ounces (one cup) of water after exercise, and continue to drink water at regular intervals throughout the day. A lactating woman who exercises should drink a minimum of 16 8 ounce glasses of water a day; that's 4 quarts or 8+ pounds of water a day. Water constitutes approximately 57% of your total body weight (Guyton, 1987).

> Lactating women secrete approximately 10 mg. of calcium per day in breast milk. However, calcium supplements do not replace this temporary loss of calcium (Kalkwarf et. al., 1999).

Chapter X
•
Aerobic Exercise

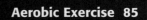

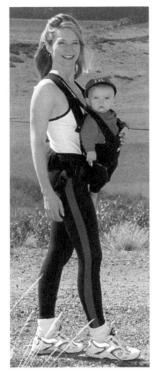

10.1 Walking with Baby in a Front Pack

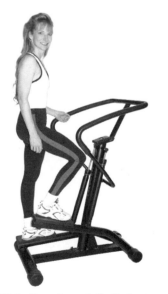

10.2 Stepping while Swinging Arms Back and Forth

Aerobic Exercise and Pregnancy

What is aerobic exercise? Aerobic exercise is exercise that strengthens your heart by maintaining your heart rate at a specific level above your resting heart rate for a specific period of time. Aerobic exercise metabolizes oxygen, which provides you with the energy to work out.

The American College of Sports Medicine recommends the following guidelines when designing an aerobic exercise program:

Frequency: perform aerobic exercise 3 – 5 times per week.

Intensity: work your heart at 60 – 90% of your maximum heart rate (please refer to Target Heart Rate).

Duration: exercise for 20 – 60 minutes.

Mode or Type: Any form of exercise that utilizes large muscles in a rhythmic manner, such as running, biking, bouncing on a ball, swimming, in-line skating, stair-stepping, etc.

In addition to the ball strengthening and stretching exercises found in this book, including aerobic exercise three to five times per week, in your regimen will further enhance your potential to burn fat, improve stamina, and strengthen your heart and lungs. Regular physical activity reduces your chances of heart disease, developing diabetes and high blood pressure, and helps build and maintain healthy bones. Furthermore, aerobic exercise promotes psychological well being and reduces feelings of depression and anxiety that are often prevalent after having a baby.

Due to all the hormonal changes of pregnancy, many women experience postpartum blues or depression. Exercise is a natural mood enhancer and can help reduce stress and depression. One study of postpartum women showed that aerobic exercise significantly decreased their total mood disturbance and significantly increased their physical vigor (Koltyn and Schultes, 1997).

Ligaments are more lax during pregnancy and postpartum due to hormonal changes. It may take 6 weeks or more for your body to balance hormone levels after delivery. During this time frame, stick with low-impact exercise, such as walking, swimming, or ball exercises, until your hormones regulate.

Walking is an excellent low-impact activity that you may start shortly after giving birth to your child. Several days after delivering my first child, I began walking short distances. These first walks would not be considered aerobic, however they helped me get stronger day by day.

Walking and jogging are two wonderful ways to exercise and get an aerobic workout, because these activities are so versatile. If you have a treadmill, you can work out indoors when the weather is poor or while your child is sleeping. Or you can have a refreshing change of pace and walk/jog outside, when weather and children permit!

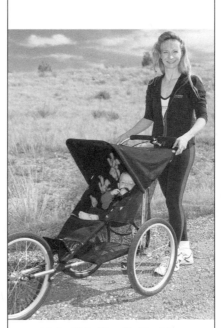

10.3 Side Handle Position

Helpful Hints

The following helpful hints were designed specifically to address exercise challenges you may encounter after having a baby.

- When walking with your baby in a front-pack, make sure you do not slouch. Raise your chest up and roll your shoulders back (see illustration 10.1). Review chapter VII on posture. If this is difficult, try adjusting the straps, pulling them tighter so that your baby sits closer to your body and higher up on your chest. This positioning will help distribute the weight more evenly, reducing the stress on your neck and shoulders.

- Carpal tunnel syndrome is common during pregnancy and after delivery due to swelling in the hands. If you experience pain in your wrists or hands and enjoy pushing a baby jogger, push the baby jogger with your hands on the sides of the handle (see illustration 10.3), or alternate pushing with the standard hand position and then the side handle position. The standard hand position for pushing the baby jogger (see illustration 10.4), tends to exacerbate carpal tunnel.

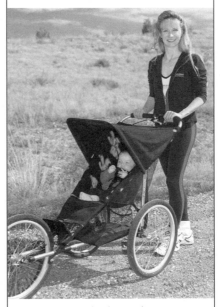

10.4 Standard Hand Position

- Alternate activities where your arms can swing freely. Arm swinging, as with walking, helps strengthen your abdominal muscles

Examples of Moderate Amounts of Activity that Promote Well-Being

More Vigorous – Less Time

Stair-climbing for 15 minutes

Shoveling snow for 15 minutes

Running 1.5 miles in 15 minutes
(10 min/mile)

Jumping rope for 15 minutes

Bicycling 4 miles in 15 minutes

Basketball (playing a game) for
15 – 20 minutes

Wheelchair basketball for 20 minutes

Swimming laps for 20 minutes

Water aerobics for 30 minutes

Walking 2 miles in 30 minutes
(15 min/mile)

Raking leaves for 30 minutes

Pushing a stroller 1.5 miles in 30 minutes

Dancing fast (social) for 30 minutes

Bicycling 5 miles in 30 minutes

Basketball (shooting baskets) for
30 minutes

Walking 1.75 miles in 35 minutes
(20 minutes/ mile)

Wheeling self in wheelchair for
30 – 40 minutes

Gardening for 30 – 45 minutes

Playing touch football for 30 – 45 minutes

Playing volleyball for 45 minutes

Washing windows or floors for
45 – 60 minutes

Washing and waxing a car for
45 – 60 minutes

Less Vigorous – More Time

*Physical Activity and Health:
A Report of the Surgeon General, 1996*

more rapidly. For instance, walk one day without pushing the baby jogger, and the next day go on a walk with the baby jogger. When using a step machine, do not rest your hands on the bar in the front of the machine, gently swing arms back and forth as you step (see illustration 10.2).

If you find that you are fatigued and overwhelmed trying to fit in aerobic workouts and meet the demands of your baby, keep in mind that the Surgeon General's Report states that "physical activity need not be strenuous to achieve health benefits." You can select any aerobic exercise or activity listed to the left that you enjoy and are able to fit into your daily life.

As the examples listed in the box show, a moderate amount of physical activity can be achieved in a variety of ways. Because the amount of activity is a function of duration, intensity, and frequency, the same amount of activity can be obtained in longer sessions of moderately intense activities (such as walking) as in shorter sessions of more strenuous activities (such as stair-climbing) – *Physical Activity and Health: A Report of the Surgeon General, 1996.*

Target Heart Rate

At rest, your heart beats slower than when you are working out. A normal resting heart rate for a female athlete may be as low as 40 to 60 beats per minute. For a moderate exerciser, the normal resting heart rate ranges from 60 to 100 beats per minute. During pregnancy, the heart beats faster and it may take four to six weeks after giving birth for your heart to return to a normal resting heart rate.

When you exercise, your heart beats faster to pump more blood to your working muscles. Since your heart is composed of muscle, it is increasingly exercised as your workout increases. With exercise, your heart muscle becomes toned, and doesn't have to beat as fast to pump the same volume of blood.

To find out if you are exercising at an intensity strong enough to benefit your heart, you will want to record your resting heart rate and then calculate your Target Heart Rate.

Note: The best time to measure your resting heart rate is in the early morning, before you get out of bed and start your activities for the day. This gives you a nice excuse to stay in bed a few minutes longer! (Refer to the section on "How to Take Your Pulse").

Calculate Your Target Heart Rate Range

First, find your Maximum Heart Rate by subtracting your age from 220

Maximum Heart Rate = 220 minus your age

Your Target Heart Rate Range should be 60% to 90% of your Maximum Heart Rate

Lower limit of Target Heart Rate = .60 x Maximum Heart Rate

Upper limit of Target Heart Rate = .90 x Maximum Heart Rate

You will want to exercise with an intensity that places you within your Target Heart Rate Range.

A normal resting heart rate for a female athlete may be as low as 40 to 60 beats per minute. For a moderate exerciser, the normal resting heart rate ranges from 60 to 100 beats per minute.

•

During pregnancy, the heart beats faster and it may take four to six weeks after giving birth for your heart to return to a normal resting heart rate.

•

With exercise, your heart muscle becomes toned, and doesn't have to beat as fast to pump the same volume of blood.

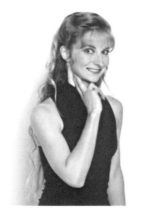

10.5 Carotid Artery Pulse

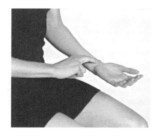

10.6 Radial Artery Pulse

Example for a 30 year old woman

Maximum Heart Rate = 220 minus 30

Maximum Heart Rate = 190 beats per minute

Lower limit of Target Heart Rate = .60 x 190

Lower limit = 114 beats per minute

Upper limit of Target Heart Rate = .90 x 190

Upper limit = 171 beats per minute

To achieve desired results, a 30 year old woman would need to exercise at an intensity that would make her heart beat at least 114 beats per minute, but not to exceed 171 beats per minute.

Note: Always check with your healthcare professional before beginning an aerobic exercise program.

How to Take Your Pulse

Measure your pulse on either the carotid artery (on your neck) (see illustration 10.5) or on your radial artery (on your wrist) (see illustration 10.6). Use your fingertips, not your thumbs. Your thumb has its own pulse, so you won't be able to get an accurate reading. Use your fingers to apply light fingertip pressure to the arteries. Anything heavier may restrict blood flow.

Find your carotid pulse by placing the tips of your index fingers and middle fingers just below the jawbone on the side of your neck.

Find your radial pulse by placing two fingers on the palm side of your wrist above the base of the thumb.

After you have found your pulse, count the beats for 10 seconds, counting the first beat as zero. For accuracy, use a stopwatch or a clock with a second hand, then multiply the number of beats you counted by six (6). This will give you your heart rate in beats per minute.

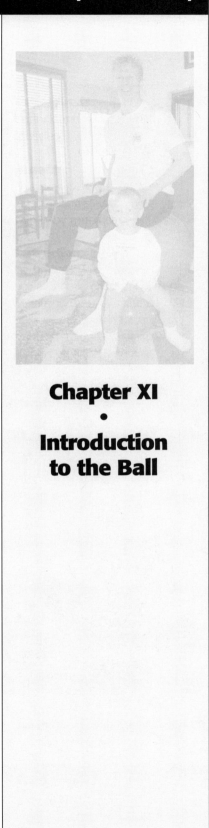

Chapter XI
·
Introduction to the Ball

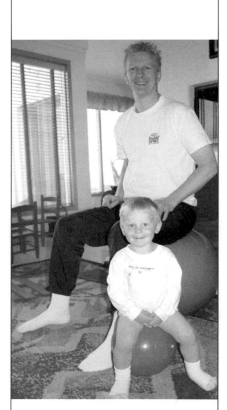

11.1 Provides entertainment for the entire family (fathers included).

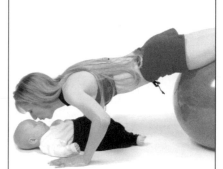

11.2 Allows you time to work out while entertaining your baby.

Why Work Out On a Ball?

Chances are you have seen brightly colored exercise balls on television, in health clubs, or physical therapy clinics. These large, inflatable vinyl balls have been used by physical therapists since the 1960's to help children improve their strength, balance, and reflexes. Now the exercise balls are not only used by physical therapists and children, but by professional athletic teams, ballet troupes, and health club members throughout the world.

You may ask yourself, why work out on a ball? In my professional experience, I have found that my clients are more likely to follow through with an exercise program if it is fun and doesn't feel like exercise. For this reason, and for the many benefits listed below, I routinely recommend ball exercises to women who have recently had a baby.

Both you and your baby will benefit from a ball workout. Listed below are many benefits to exercising on the ball.

Benefits to Mom

• Provides a total body stretching and strengthening workout: abdomen, back, buttocks, chest, inner and outer thighs, legs, pelvic floor muscles, shoulders, and neck.

• Increases your metabolism and helps you lose weight.

• Improves your mood.

• Reduces stress, anxiety, and depression.

• Relieves muscle tension by increasing circulation to tight muscles.

• Strengthens bones by improving bone mineral content and helping to prevent osteoporosis.

• Provides a low-impact workout that does not cause undue stress on individual body parts.

- Requires inexpensive equipment and can be done in the privacy of your home.

- Improves posture, body awareness, and self-image.

- Helps align the spine and nourish the discs in the back through the bouncing movements.

- Provides entertainment for the entire family (fathers included) (see illustration 11.1).

- Allows you time to workout while entertaining your baby (see illustration 11.2).

- Re-energizes your body.

Benefits to Baby

- Improves baby's strength (see illustration 11.3).

- Reduces colic symptoms by bouncing baby on ball.

- Rhythmic bouncing provides a wonderful way to put your baby to sleep.

- Improves baby's balance.

- Offers an excellent way to interact socially with mom.

- Reinforces the importance of exercise by introducing your child to exercise at a young age (see illustration 11.4).

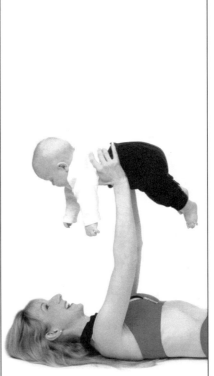

11.3 Improves baby's strength.

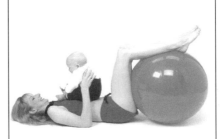

11.4 Reinforces the importance of exercise by introducing your child to exercise at a young age.

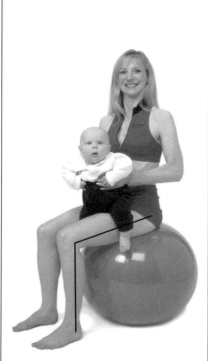

11.5 Ideal Ball Size

How to Determine Appropriate Ball Size

Once you have decided to begin a ball exercise routine, you will need to determine what ball size is appropriate for you. Ideally, when you sit on the ball, you will want your feet flat, knees shoulder-width apart, and hips even with or higher than your knees (see illustration 11.5).

Ball size is not only determined by your height, but also by your weight and exercise goal. If you are 5' 6" (168 centimeters) tall, and weigh 125 pounds (47 kilograms), I recommend you use a 55 centimeter ball. However, if you are 5' 6" tall and weigh 180 pounds (67 kilograms), a 65 centimeter ball may be more appropriate. If you are 5' 6" (168 centimeters) tall and have very long legs, you also may want to use a 65 centimeter ball.

What can you do if you are 5' 3" tall (160 centimeters) and purchased a book and ball package, and the ball is 65 centimeters? Don't inflate your ball as much. Typically, it is better to go up a ball size than to go down a ball size. Inflate your ball in the same manner as instructed in the *Step-by-Step Guide to Inflating Your Ball*. Your ball will not be as firm as a fully inflated 55 centimeter ball, but you will gain the same benefits.

The following chart serves as a guideline for determining the appropriate ball size:

Ball Sizes	Heights
30 cm. ball (14 inches)	for use with children 1 – 2 years
45 cm. ball (18 inches)	<152 cm. or <5' 0" tall
55 cm. ball (22 inches)	152 – 170 cm. or 5' 0" – 5' 7" tall
65 cm. ball (26 inches)	171 – 183 cm. or 5' 8' – 6' 3" tall
75 cm. ball (30 inches)	>183 cm. or >6' 3" tall

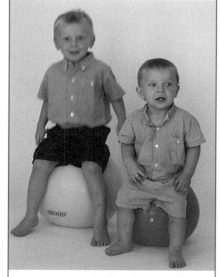

11.6 45 cm. Ball and 30 cm. Ball

Proper Inflation Techniques

The question I am most frequently asked is, "How do I inflate the exercise ball?" The six pieces of equipment listed below are the most practical. I do not recommend inflating a ball by mouth or with a bicycle pump, since both of these inflation methods require an extensive amount of time and energy. I recommend the air compressor, because it takes the least amount of time and effort to blow up the ball.

1. air compressor
2. hand pump
3. foot pump
4. raft pump
5. air mattress pump
6. gas station air pump with a trigger nozzle adapter

The following is a **Step-by-Step Guide to Inflating Your Ball**:
• Allow the ball to reach room temperature.
• Determine the size of your ball by rotating it until you find a number. This number is the recommended ball height (diameter).
• Put a pencil mark on the wall at the specified ball height.
• Remove the plug from your ball.
• Insert pump nozzle into opening of ball.
• Using good body mechanics, inflate the ball <u>up to</u> or <u>slightly below</u> the pencil mark (see illustration 11.7).
• Withdraw pump nozzle from ball.
• Place plug back in ball.

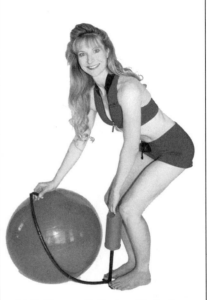

11.7 **Proper Inflation Technique with Hand Pump**

Every three to four months the exercise balls may require additional air. If you use your ball extensively, you may need to add air even more frequently.

If your ball leaks air and it is difficult to ascertain the location of the leak, place the ball in the bathtub. You will be able to identify the leak by looking for air bubbles. If you find the ball is leaking around the plug, obtain a new plug and place it in the ball. (Most ball manufacturers package the balls with a second plug). If you are unable to prevent the ball from leaking, it may be time to purchase another one. Patch kits are not available for the balls.

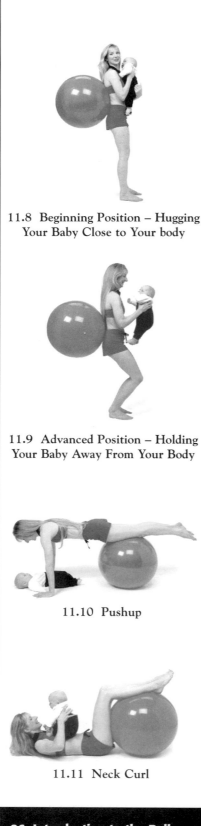

11.8 Beginning Position – Hugging Your Baby Close to Your body

11.9 Advanced Position – Holding Your Baby Away From Your Body

11.10 Pushup

11.11 Neck Curl

Ball Exercise Tips

- Perform ball exercises only after you have mastered the core stability exercises as illustrated in the Core Strengthening chapter. Vera-Garcia, et. al. (2000), found that performing a sit up on the ball increased abdominal muscle activity and changed the way the muscles worked together to stabilize the spine as compared to a traditional sit up. They suggest these findings imply a higher demand is placed on the motor (muscle) system when performing ball exercises.

- Always perform exercises without your baby first. Hold your baby only if you are able to perform the exercise safely without any undue risk to you or your child.

- Hug your baby close to your body, as in illustration 11.8. This will place less stress on your abdomen, arms, and back. Holding your baby away from your body, as in illustration 11.9, may make the exercise too difficult.

- The closer the ball is to the body, the easier it is to maintain a neutral spine and perform the exercise. For example, to make the pushup easier, roll the ball closer to your hands, to make the exercise more difficult, roll the ball toward your feet (see illustration 11.10).

- Never hold your breath when performing an exercise. Always exhale when the exercise is most difficult. Exhale as you perform a *Neck Curl*, as depicted, and inhale as you return your head to the floor (see illustration 11.11).

- Avoid bouncing on the ball if it causes incontinence. The bouncing motion may exacerbate your symptoms.

- Perform exercises away from furniture and sharp objects.

- The following may puncture an exercise ball: sharp objects (belt buckles, jewelry, staples, cat claws etc.), heat sources (direct sunlight, heaters, fireplaces, etc.), and inflating the ball beyond the maximum diameter.

- If at any time an exercise causes discomfort or pain, revise your exercise regimen by reducing intensity, frequency, duration, and/or type of exercise. If any of these symptoms persist, discontinue the exercise.

Chapter XII
•
Stretching Exercises

To properly stretch a muscle, maintain a slow, static stretch. Bouncing or sudden stretching of a muscle triggers a reflex contraction in the muscle being stretched. This contraction is referred to as the myotactic reflex or stretch reflex.

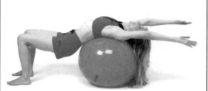

12.1 Abdominal and Back Stretch

Stretching Basics

In our present day society, it is difficult not to become caught up in a fast paced, busy lifestyle that predisposes us to stress and muscle tension. Tension builds up in our muscles while driving, talking on the phone, or sitting at a computer terminal. These activities cause individual muscle fibers to shorten, decreasing flexibility, and increasing the likelihood of injury.

Stretching exercises relieve stress, improve posture, and increase flexibility in tight muscles. Stretching techniques are not complicated, yet there is definitely a proper and improper way to stretch.

To properly stretch a muscle, maintain a slow, static stretch. Bouncing or sudden stretching of a muscle triggers a reflex contraction in the muscle being stretched. This contraction is referred to as the **myotactic reflex** or **stretch reflex**. The stretch reflex protects our muscles from being overstretched or injured. Bouncing while stretching is therefore counterproductive and may lead to your muscle being overstretched or injured. Watch your cat or dog, they stretch in a slow, sustained motion without any bouncing!

Proper stretching techniques are essential to effectively increase the length of the muscle and surrounding tissue. Stretching exercises should be performed 15 – 20 minutes before exercising and once again thereafter.

The following guidelines are adapted from "The Warm Up Procedure: To Stretch or Not to Stretch. A Brief Review" by Craig Smith.

1. Avoid Bouncing.
2. Slowly stretch into level of tolerance, not pain.
3. Do not hold your breath. Exhale while stretching.
4. Hold stretch for 15 – 20 seconds.
5. Release stretch slowly.
6. Repeat stretch 3 times.
7. Repeat stretch on both sides of the body.

Stretching Exercises

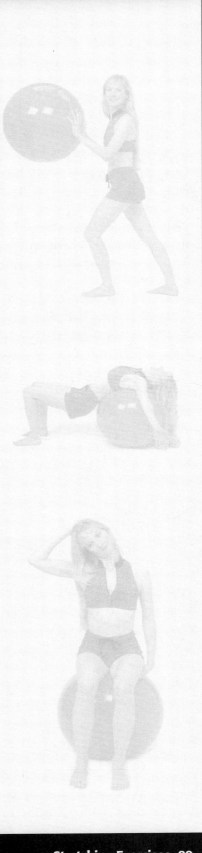

Target Area:
Side neck muscles.

Benefits:
When breast or bottle-feeding, the shoulders tend to creep up toward the ears causing tightness in the neck muscles and neck discomfort. This exercise reduces neck tension and improves posture by stretching your side neck muscles.

Instruction:
Sit on ball with feet shoulder-width apart. Sit on left hand. Tilt head toward right shoulder. Place right hand on head and gently pull head on shoulder. Repeat on opposite side.

Helpful Hints:
• Avoid arching back.
• Neutral spine: A position where back is not arched or flat, it is somewhere in between.

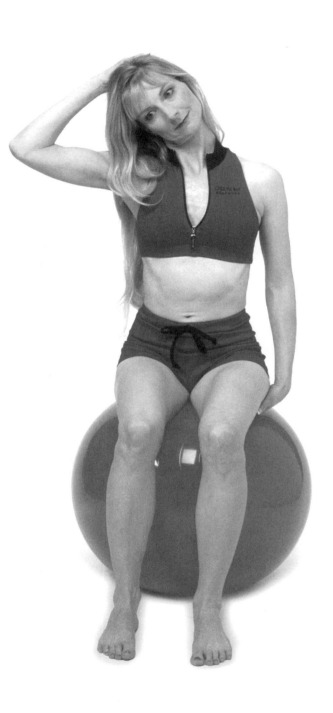

Hold:
15 – 20 seconds

Repeat:
3 – 5 times

Frequency:
2 times per week

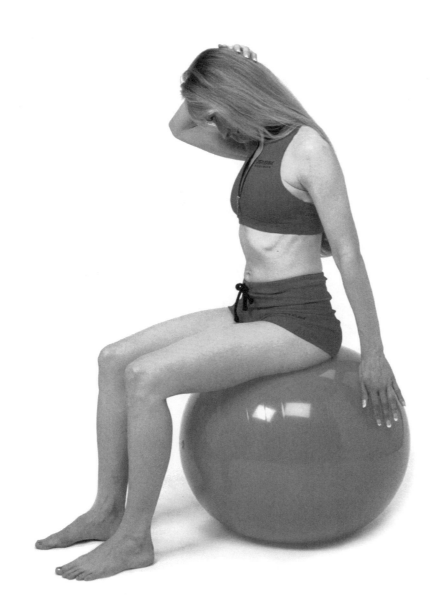

Target Areas:
Back of neck and upper shoulder blade muscles.

Benefits:
When breast or bottle-feeding, the shoulders tend to creep up toward the ears causing tightness in the neck muscles and neck discomfort. This exercise reduces neck tension and improves posture by stretching your neck and upper shoulder blade muscles. It stretches the muscles most likely to cause neck and shoulder tension.

Instruction:
Sit on ball with feet shoulder-width apart. Place right hand behind head. Bend neck forward and look down at right knee. Extend left arm slightly behind back and reach for floor. Repeat on opposite side.

Helpful Hints:
• Avoid arching back.
• Neutral spine: A position where back is not arched or flat, it is somewhere in between.

Hold:
15 – 20 seconds

Repeat:
3 – 5 times

Frequency:
2 times per week

Front of Wrist Stretch

★★☆☆☆

Target Area:
Front of wrist muscles.

Benefits:
Newborns and babies with colic get a lot of back patting. This repetitive patting action, and repeatedly lifting baby throughout the day may cause the wrists to become sore. This stretch improves range of motion at the wrist, and helps alleviate wrist soreness.

Instruction:
Kneel. Lie with abdomen on ball. Place hands in front of ball with palms down. Gently roll ball forward so that shoulders are in front of wrists. Hold, then gently roll ball backward to starting position.

Helpful Hints:
• Avoid hyperextending elbows.
• If you have carpal tunnel syndrome, try stretching wrists in a non-weight bearing position, such as sitting.

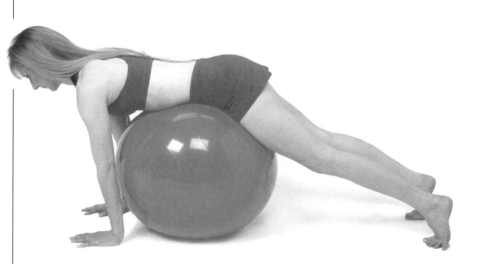

Hold:
15 – 20 seconds

Repeat:
3 – 5 times

Frequency:
2 times per week

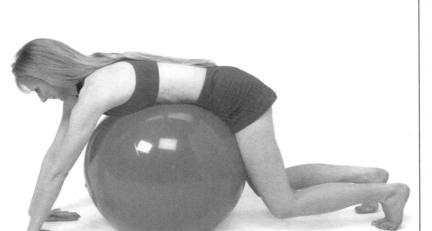

Target Area:
Back of wrist muscles.

Benefits:
Newborns and babies with colic get a lot of back patting. This repetitive patting action, and repeatedly lifting baby throughout the day may cause the wrists to become sore. This stretch improves range of motion at the wrist and helps alleviate wrist soreness.

Instruction:
Kneel. Lie with abdomen on ball. Place hands in front of ball with back of hands touching floor, and fingers pointing toward ball. Gently roll ball backward so that shoulders are behind wrists. Try to keep back of hands on floor. Hold, then gently roll ball forward to starting position.

Helpful Hints:
• Avoid hyperextending elbows.
• If you have carpal tunnel syndrome, try stretching wrists in a non-weight bearing position, such as sitting.

Hold:	**Repeat:**	**Frequency:**
15 – 20 seconds	3 – 5 times	2 times per week

Shoulder Stretch

★ ☆ ☆ ☆ ☆

Target Area:
Shoulder muscles.

Benefits:
Lifting and holding baby requires the shoulder muscles to work overtime causing shoulder tension. This stretch improves shoulder flexibility, preventing neck and shoulder pain.

Instruction:
Kneel. Place ball in front of body and hands on ball. Lean forward and roll ball away from body. Lower head so ears are between straight arms.

Helpful Hint:
• Place a towel under knees if you experience knee discomfort caused by a hard surface.

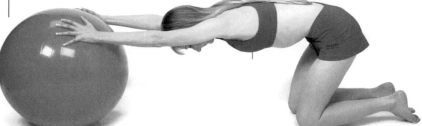

Hold:	**Repeat:**	**Frequency:**
15 – 20 seconds	3 – 5 times	2 times per week

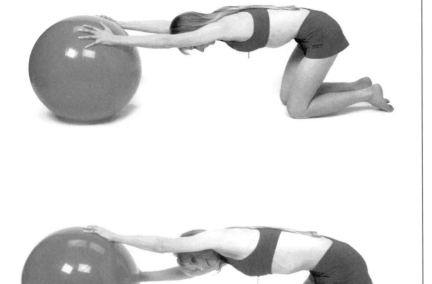

Target Areas:
Shoulder and side trunk muscles.

Benefits:
When holding your baby on your hip (right handed women tend to hold baby on left hip) we tend to hike up this hip and raise the shoulder on the same side. This exercise stretches the shoulder and trunk muscles, preventing shoulder, back, and hip pain.

Instruction:
Kneel. Place hands on ball. Roll ball away from body. Keep hands on ball. Keep ears between straight arms. Roll ball from side to side. Hold stretch on each side of body.

Helpful Hint:
• Place a towel under knees if you experience knee discomfort caused by a hard surface.

Hold:	**Repeat:**	**Frequency:**
15 – 20 seconds	3 – 5 times	2 times per week

Nerve Stretch

★★☆☆☆

Target Areas:
Nerves and muscles in upper body, shoulder, and chest muscles.

Benefits:
To stretch nerves in upper body, shoulder, and chest muscles. This exercise helps prevent carpal tunnel and thoracic outlet syndrome, a condition caused by compressed nerves and vessels in the neck and arm region.

Instruction:
Stand with feet shoulder-width apart. Place ball between wall and right hand. Extend wrist back so palm of hand touches ball. Rotate head in the opposite direction. Keep shoulders down. Repeat on opposite side.

Helpful Hint:
• Keep hips straight, and avoid rotating them when turning head.

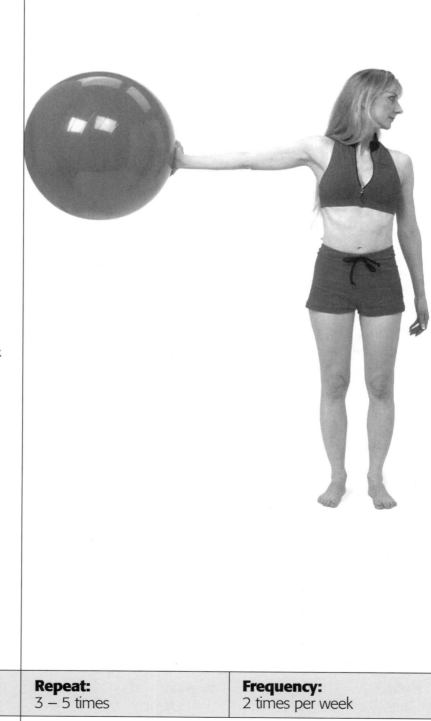

Hold:
15 – 30 seconds

Repeat:
3 – 5 times

Frequency:
2 times per week

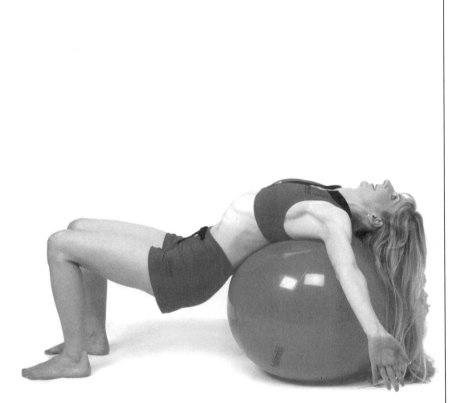

Target Areas:
Chest, arm, and finger muscles.

Benefits:
Pregnancy, breast and bottle-feeding, lifting, and holding baby all require carrying additional weight in front of the body. These activities cause the shoulders to droop, and the back to round. This exercise is a wonderful way to improve posture by stretching the chest, arm, and finger muscles.

Instruction:
Sit on ball. Place hands on ball. Walk feet out so head and shoulders rest on ball. Lower buttocks toward ball. Raise arms out away from body. Find the position that stretches chest, arms, and fingers the most by slowly moving arms up and down. Extend wrists back and straighten fingers. Hold, then gently roll back to starting position.

Helpful Hint:
• Always keep head supported by ball. If your head is unable to reach ball comfortably, place a small pillow under your head.

Hold:	**Repeat:**	**Frequency:**
15 – 20 seconds	3 – 5 times	2 times per week

Target Areas:
Abdominal and back muscles.

Benefits:
Breast and bottle feeding, and holding babies in front of the body tends to makes us slouch. This exercise improves posture by stretching the abdominal and back muscles in the opposite direction of the slouch.

Instruction:
Sit on ball. Place hands on side of ball. Walk feet out away from ball so head and shoulders rest on ball. Lower buttocks toward ball. Raise arms overhead. Hold, then relax arms and repeat.

Helpful Hints:
• Advanced Abdominal and Back Stretch: Follow directions as above. Raise arms overhead and straighten legs (equivalent to ★★★).
• Always keep head supported by ball. If your head is unable to reach ball comfortably, place a small pillow under your head.

Hold:	Repeat:	Frequency:
15 – 20 seconds	3 – 5 times	2 times per week

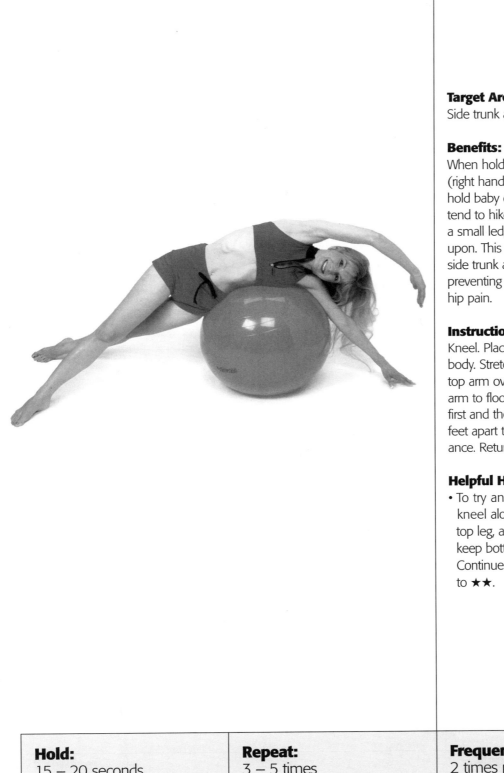

Target Areas:
Side trunk and shoulder muscles.

Benefits:
When holding baby on hip (right handed women tend to hold baby on left hip), women tend to hike up the hip to provide a small ledge for the baby to rest upon. This exercise stretches the side trunk and shoulder muscles preventing shoulder, back, and hip pain.

Instruction:
Kneel. Place ball alongside body. Stretch over ball raising top arm overhead and bottom arm to floor. Straighten top leg first and then bottom leg. Split feet apart to provide better balance. Return to kneeling position.

Helpful Hint:
• To try an easier side stretch, kneel alongside ball. Straighten top leg, as above, however keep bottom knee bent. Continue as above. Equivalent to ★★.

Hold:	**Repeat:**	**Frequency:**
15 – 20 seconds	3 – 5 times	2 times per week

Target Area:
Lower back muscles.

Benefits:
Due, in part, to tightness in the lower back muscles, the arched back, pregnant-look is still common after baby is born. This exercise improves posture and reduces lower back tension by gently stretching these lower back muscles.

Instruction:
Lie on back with legs on ball. Raise and place baby on top of legs. Hold onto baby's hands, arms, or torso. Bend knees to chest.

Helpful Hint:
• Always try exercise without baby first (equivalent to ★).

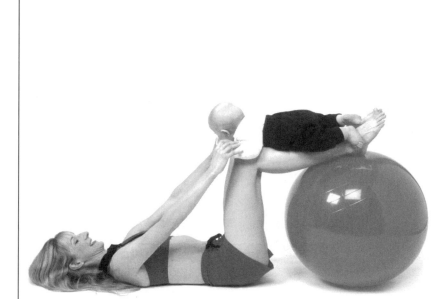

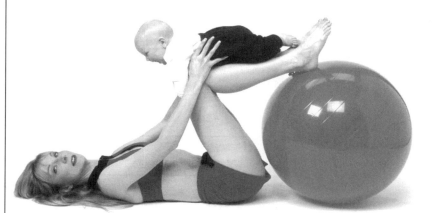

Hold:	**Repeat:**	**Frequency:**
15 – 20 seconds	3 – 5 times	2 times per week

Target Area:
Buttock muscles.

Benefits:
Extra weight and swelling can cause discomfort in the buttock region. This stretch improves flexibility and circulation in the buttocks.

Instruction:
Kneel. Place both palms on ball in front of body. Stretch arms out straight. Extend one leg back. Lean forward as ball is pushed forward. Repeat with opposite leg.

Helpful Hint:
• Avoid performing this exercise if you have knee pain.

Hold:	**Repeat:**	**Frequency:**
15 – 20 seconds	3 – 5 times	2 times per week

Target Areas:
Front thigh and hip muscles.

Benefits:
During pregnancy, most of the abdominal weight gained is in the front of the body, causing the lower back to arch and tightness in the front hip and thigh muscles. This exercise improves posture and hip alignment.

Instruction:
Sit on ball. Place baby on right knee. Slide left leg behind ball and straighten. Keep front leg bent. Rotate body toward baby. Maintain a neutral spine. Repeat with opposite side.

Helpful Hints:
• Avoid arching back. If you arch your back, you will not feel the stretch in your front thigh and hip muscles.
• Neutral spine: A position where the back is not arched or flat, it is somewhere in between.

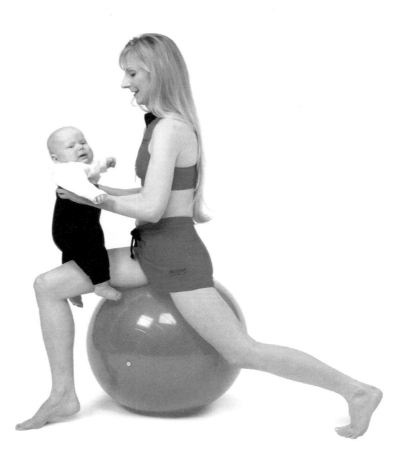

Hold:
15 – 20 seconds

Repeat:
3 – 5 times

Frequency:
2 times per week

Target Area:
Back of leg muscles.

Benefits:
The sitting position, as with feeding, holding, or snuggling with your baby, causes the back leg muscles to tighten. This exercise stretches the back leg muscles and helps prevent or ease low back pain.

Instruction:
Lie on back and place calves on ball. Place hands behind right knee. Straighten right knee and pull toes down toward nose. Return to starting position. Repeat with opposite side.

Helpful Hint:
• Avoid pulling knee to chest

Hold:	**Repeat:**	**Frequency:**
15 – 20 seconds	3 – 5 times	2 times per week

★☆☆☆☆

Target Area:
Large calf muscles.

Benefits:
Rocking baby in a rocking chair and bouncing baby on the knees strengthens calf muscles but also tightens them. This exercise stretches calf muscles and decreases cramping in calf muscles.

Instruction:
Stand with feet shoulder-width apart. Place ball between wall and hands. Bend left knee. Straighten right knee behind body. Keep knees aligned over feet. Return to starting position. Repeat with opposite side.

Helpful Hints:
• To stretch appropriate muscles, avoid turning feet. Keep toes pointing toward wall.
• Keep heels on floor.

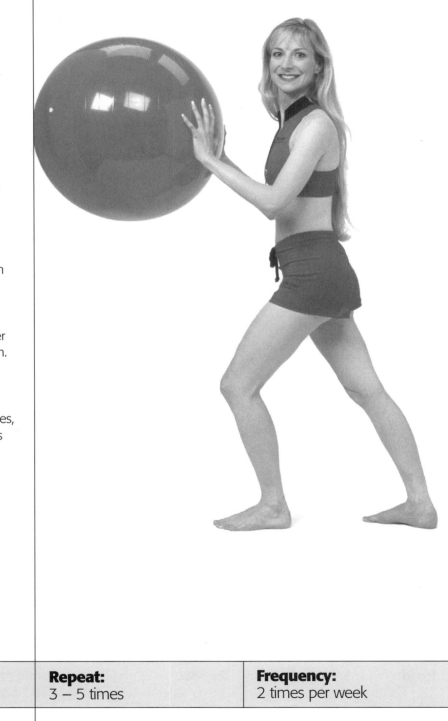

Hold:	**Repeat:**	**Frequency:**
15 – 20 seconds	3 – 5 times	2 times per week

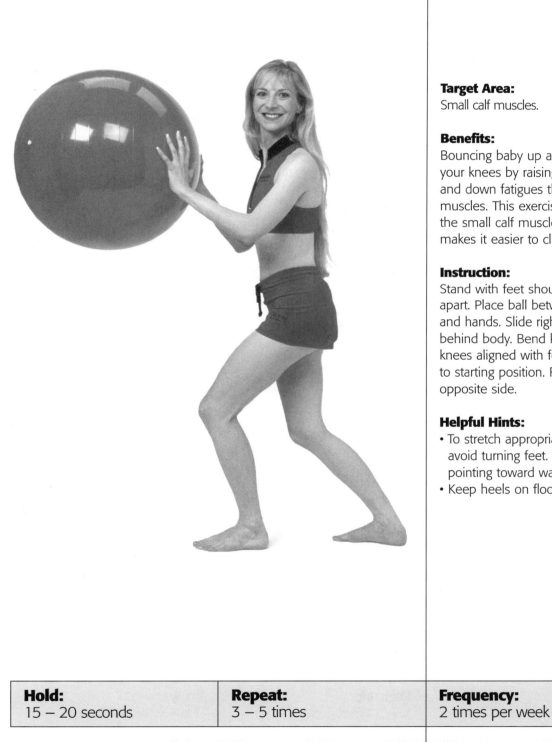

Target Area:
Small calf muscles.

Benefits:
Bouncing baby up and down on your knees by raising heels up and down fatigues the small calf muscles. This exercise stretches the small calf muscles and makes it easier to climb stairs.

Instruction:
Stand with feet shoulder-width apart. Place ball between wall and hands. Slide right knee behind body. Bend knees. Keep knees aligned with feet. Return to starting position. Repeat with opposite side.

Helpful Hints:
• To stretch appropriate muscles, avoid turning feet. Keep toes pointing toward wall.
• Keep heels on floor.

Hold:	**Repeat:**	**Frequency:**
15 – 20 seconds	3 – 5 times	2 times per week

Shin and Front Foot Stretch

★☆☆☆☆

Target Areas:
Shin and front foot muscles.

Benefits:
Rocking baby in a rocker and walking or jogging on hard surfaces can cause shin splints or pain in the shins. This exercise prevents shin splints or helps reduce shin discomfort.

Instruction:
Stand with feet shoulder-width apart. Place ball between wall and hands. Place foot behind body with top of foot touching floor. Press top of foot into floor. Return to starting position. Repeat with opposite side.

Hold:	Repeat:	Frequency:
15 – 20 seconds	3 – 5 times	2 times per week

Chapter XIII
•
Strengthening Exercises

The American College of Sports Medicine (ACSM), 1990, recommends that a minimum of 8 to 10 resistive exercises be performed at least two times per week using major muscle groups. Each exercise should include a minimum of one set with 8 to 12 repetitions.

•

Regardless of recommended repetitions in this book, or by the ACSM, you must decide how many repetitions and sets are best for you by following the established guidelines in this book.

Strengthening Basics

The American College of Sports Medicine (ACSM), 1990, recommends that a minimum of 8 to 10 resistive exercises be performed at least two times per week using major muscle groups. Each exercise should include a minimum of one set with 8 to 12 repetitions. Ball strengthening exercises are considered a resistive exercise, since your body weight is used as the resistance.

Strengthening exercises should be preceded by a 5 – 10 minute low-intensity warm-up, followed by stretching exercises, and a 5 minute cool down. Stretching exercises should be performed 15 – 20 minutes before exercising and once again thereafter (Smith, 1994). Warm-up and cool down activities may include a variety of activities – walking, bouncing on the ball while swinging your arms, jumping jacks on the ball, or pushing your child in a stroller. For further warm-up and cool down ideas, refer to the mini-workout chapter.

Repetitions

How many repetitions (reps), or times, should an exercise be performed? The ACSM recommends you perform each exercise 8 to 12 times. However, remember that the ASCM recommendations are only guidelines.

The bottom line is, before you can increase the number of repetitions, the quality of your exercise must be good. When your body begins to fatigue, it causes you to substitute or use the incorrect muscles to perform an exercise. For instance, if you are performing the Back and Neck Strengthener exercise on page 147, and you are able to perform 6 repetitions before fatigue and on the 7th repetition you begin to arch your back or raise your leg too high, then it is time to stop. You would have a 6 repetition maximum (6 RM) for this exercise. Regardless of recommended repetitions in this book, or by the ACSM, you must decide how many repetitions and sets are best for you by following the guidelines established in this book.

"Most studies have found that RMs that allow for six or fewer repetitions (i.e., low RMs) provide the most strength and power benefits, that weights (ball strengthening exercises) based on 6 RM–12 RM provide moderate strength, power, and endurance gains; and that weights based on RMs of 20 and above provide primarily muscular endurance gains with no strength gain." (Baechle, 1994, pg. 442).

These studies were performed on healthy athletes, not with women who have just had a baby. I frequently recommend less than 6 repetitions for specific exercises throughout the book. I believe postpartum women need to begin with fewer repetitions at the initiation of an exercise program due to weakness and the physical changes their bodies have undergone in the previous nine months. Repetitions can always be increased as the body becomes stronger.

Sets

What is a set? A set is a specific number of repetitions completed without a rest break. If the recommended repetitions for a specific exercise are 8, then you would perform 8 repetitions in each set. When first beginning an exercise program, I recommend you perform one set of each exercise and progress to two sets when you are able to maintain good form throughout all repetitions.

Rest

A brief rest period is recommended between each exercise set and between different exercises. This rest period allows your muscles time to recuperate for the next set or exercise. How long should a rest period be between sets and different exercises? A standard rest period of 30 to 60 seconds (Baechle, 1994) is to be used between sets and exercises in this book, unless otherwise noted. As your fitness level improves, you may begin decreasing the rest period to 15 seconds. The following is a good rule of thumb for deciding when to decrease your rest period: when your heart rate returns to 100 to 110 beats per minute and you are able to maintain good form with a reduced rest period.

Frequency

As stated previously, the ACSM recommends that resistive training be performed at least two times per week. Ball strengthening exercises may be performed in one longer session per day or several brief sessions per day. When performing one-star and two-star exercises, you may perform them every day. However, when you begin doing

---

When first beginning an exercise program, I recommend you perform one set of each exercise and progress to two sets when you are able to maintain good form throughout all repetitions.

·

A standard rest period of 30 to 60 seconds (Baechle, 1994) is to be used between sets and exercises in this book, unless otherwise noted. As your fitness level improves, you may begin decreasing the rest period to 15 seconds.

·

When performing one-star and two-star exercises, you may perform them every day. However, when you begin doing three, four, and five-star exercises, it is best to alternate days you perform the exercises.

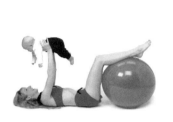

13.1 Baby Press

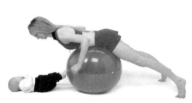

13.2 Shoulder Rowing

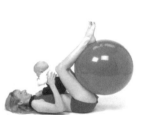

13.3 Lower Abdominal Crunch

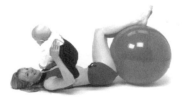

13.4 Knee Rolls

three, four, and five-star exercises, it is best to alternate days you perform the exercises. For example, strengthen your upper body and abdominal muscles on Monday, Wednesday, and Friday, and strengthen the lower body and back on Tuesday, Thursday, and Saturday.

Sequence of Exercises

Exercise sequence is dependent upon muscle size, which areas of the body are weak, and your exercise goal. Weak or small muscles tend to fatigue more quickly, so they should be placed at the beginning of an exercise regimen. These muscles should be exercised more frequently with a greater number of repetitions. If your goal is to work out in the least amount of time with the greatest benefits, then the following exercise sequencing techniques are of benefit.

Supersetting involves exercising two opposing body parts with a minimal rest break between exercises. Circuit training is a form of superset exercises. For example, you would perform a biceps curl followed by a triceps press. Or, perform a Baby Press (see illustration 13.1) followed by Shoulder Rowing (see illustration 13.2). Supersetting allows opposing muscle groups more time to recuperate than with compound or pre-exhaustion techniques, since there is a greater rest period between exercises for the same muscle groups.

Compound setting entails exercising one muscle group with two different exercises in an alternating manner. This mode of exercising is more intense than supersetting. For example, you would perform a sit up followed by a diagonal sit up. Or perform a Lower Abdominal Crunch (see illustration 13.3) followed by Knee Rolls (see illustration 13.4).

Pre-exhaustion is a technique used to focus on strengthening one muscle followed with an exercise that targets many muscles. This mode of exercise is also more intense than supersetting. For example, you would perform a biceps curl followed by a power clean. Or, perform a Sitting Squat (see illustration 13.5) followed by a Standing Squat (see illustration 13.6).

Supersetting, compound setting, and pre-exhaustion techniques require you to be in much better shape than when you perform just a few exercises. However, they add variety to the workout and provide greater strength gains in less time (Baechle, 1994). For ideas on how to implement these techniques, please refer to Mini-Workouts in Chapter XIV.

Flow Chart

I have provided a flow chart at the end of the book so that you may record your progress on the number of sets and repetitions of each exercise completed, along with your exercise heart rate. The example below shows you how to fill out the flow chart correctly. By recording your sets, repetitions, and heart rate, you can follow your weekly progress at a glance. If you are unfamiliar with taking your pulse to calculate your exercise heart rate, please refer to How to Take Your Pulse on page 90.

Follow the guidelines in this chapter, take time to smile at your baby, and enjoy the exercises!

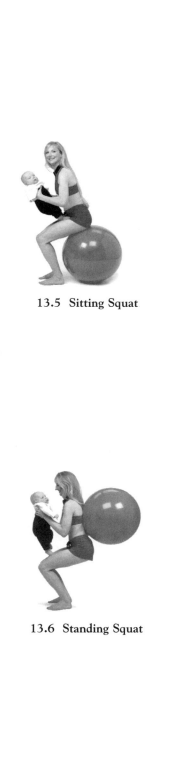

13.5 Sitting Squat

13.6 Standing Squat

FLOW CHART

Date: / Exercise:	Set	Hold Time	1	2	3	Exercise Heart Rate	Hold Time	1	2	3	Exercise Heart Rate	Hold Time	1	2	3	Exercise Heart Rate	Hold Time	1	2	3	Exercise Heart Rate	Hold Time	1	2	3	Exercise Heart Rate
Chest and Finger Stretch	Rep	20	3	-	-	100																				
Transverse Abdominis	Rep	5	5	5	-	-																				
Airplane	Rep	-	8	8	-	140																				
	Rep																									
	Rep																									
	Rep																									
	Rep																									
	Rep																									
	Rep																									
	Rep																									
	Rep																									
	Rep																									
	Rep																									
	Rep																									
	Rep																									
	Rep																									
	Rep																									
	Rep																									
	Rep																									
	Rep																									
	Rep																									
	Rep																									
	Rep																									
	Rep																									
	Rep																									
	Rep																									
	Rep																									

Strengthening Exercises

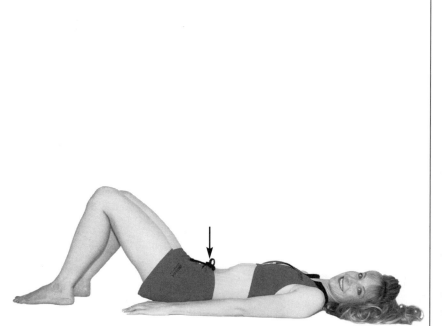

Target Areas:
Deep abdominal muscles located on the side and front of abdomen, pelvic floor, and deep lower back muscles.

Benefits:
After having a baby, a corset-like abdominal muscle (transverse abdominis) becomes very weak, predisposing a woman to poor posture, and back and pelvic pain. This exercise improves posture, strengthens abdominal and back muscles, and stabilizes the spine. It strengthens the transverse abdominis muscles with gravity. You may begin performing this exercise within 24 hours after giving birth.

Instruction:
Maintain a neutral spine position. Take a relaxed breath in and out. Now without breathing in, slowly and gently draw the lower abdomen in towards the spine. Hold, breathe lightly. The upper abdomen moves with light breathing. Relax the abdomen gradually.

Helpful Hints:
• This is a very gentle exercise. If you pull lower abdomen in too far, internal oblique muscles will be recruited.
• Avoid movement of the trunk or pelvis, and avoid using inner thigh and buttock muscles.
• If you find this exercise difficult to do, try a Transverse Abdominis Raise which is performed on hands and knees.
• This exercise may be performed lying down, standing, and later while sitting.
• Neutral spine: refer to page 41.

Hold:
5 – 20 seconds

Repeat:
2 – 10 times

Frequency: 2 – 3 times per day, just before you get out of bed, or as tolerated

Target Areas:
Deep abdominal muscles located on the side and front of the abdomen, pelvic floor, and deep lower back muscles.

Benefits:
After having a baby, the transverse abdominis, a corset-like muscle of the abdomen, becomes very weak predisposing a woman to poor posture, and back and pelvic pain. This exercise improves posture, abdominal and pelvic floor strength, helps stabilize the spine, and strengthens the transverse abdominis muscle against gravity.

Instruction:
Kneel. Lean forward and place hands on floor. Align shoulders and hands, and hips and knees. Maintain head alignment with body, and a neutral spine position. Take a relaxed breath in and out. Now without breathing in, slowly and gently draw the lower abdomen in towards the spine. Hold, breathe lightly. Relax the abdomen gradually.

Helpful Hints:
• This is a very gentle exercise. If you pull lower abdomen up too far, internal oblique muscles will be recruited.
• This exercise may be performed lying down, standing and later while sitting.
• Avoid movement of the trunk or pelvis and avoid using inner thigh and buttock muscles.
• If you find this exercise difficult to do, perform it while lying on your back or on your abdomen.
• Neutral spine: A position where the back is not arched or flat, it is somewhere in between.

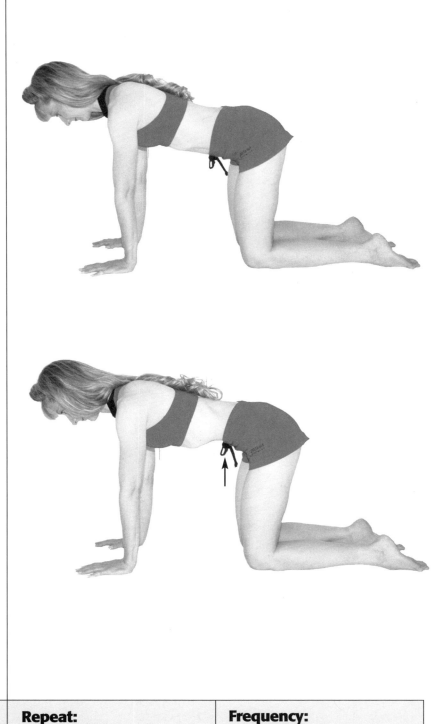

Hold:
5 – 20 seconds

Repeat:
2 – 10 times

Frequency:
2 – 3 times per day, or every time the phone rings.

Target Areas:
Deep back and deep abdominal muscles.

Benefits:
Deep back muscles should work in unison with deep abdominal muscles (transverse abdominis) to stabilize or support your trunk. Pregnancy and childbirth can cause weakness and disharmony between these muscles. This is a beginning exercise that teaches one way to properly strengthen these muscles, and can be performed within 24 hours after giving birth.

Instruction:
Lie on back with knees bent and feet shoulder-width apart. Maintain a neutral spine position by gently drawing lower abdomen in toward spine. Now **imagine** swelling out the lower back on each side of the spine. Hold, breathe lightly. Relax the back and abdomen gradually.

Helpful Hints:
• Avoid movement of trunk, pelvis, inner thighs, and buttock muscles, or bearing down when performing exercise.
• If it is difficult to feel deep back muscles tighten during this exercise, try performing this exercise on your stomach and have someone place their fingers on each side of the back bone. Feel your back muscles swell into the fingers.
• Neutral spine: A position where back is not arched or flat, it is somewhere in between.

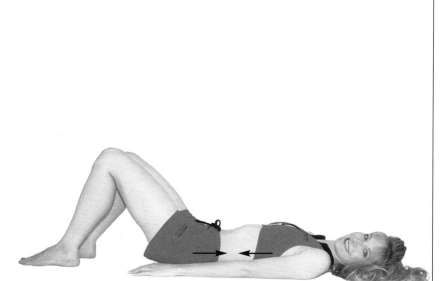

Hold:
5 – 20 seconds

Repeat:
2 – 10 times

Frequency: 2 – 3 times per day, just before getting out of bed or as tolerated.

Target Areas:
Mid-layer abdominal muscles located on sides of abdomen, and pelvic floor muscles.

Benefits:
After having a baby, external and internal oblique muscles become very weak. This exercise will teach you how to focus on contracting your obliques and pelvic floor muscles.

Instruction:
Maintain a neutral spine position. Take a relaxed breath in, and as you exhale, slowly exhale through your teeth and say SSSSSSS (abdomen should be drawn in further with this exercise than with transverse abdominis exercise). Your waist should narrow and diaphragm muscle should engage. Hold, breathe lightly. Relax sides of abdomen gradually.

Helpful Hints:
- The pelvic floor should tighten and not bulge with this exercise.
- Avoid movement of the trunk or pelvis and avoid using inner thigh and buttock muscles when performing exercise.
- Neutral spine: A position where back is not arched or flat, it is somewhere in between.

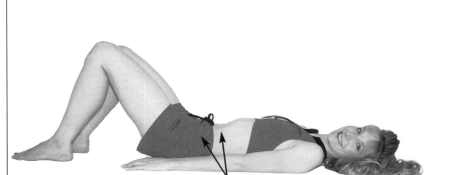

Hold:	**Repeat:**	**Frequency:**
5 – 20 seconds	2 – 10 times	2 – 3 times per day

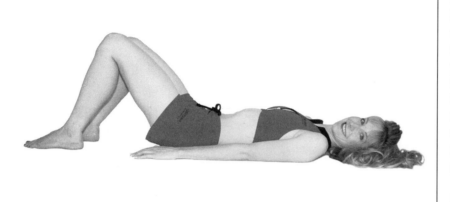

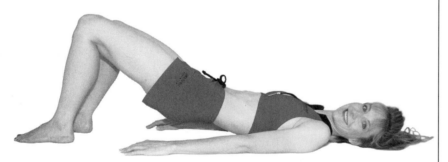

Target Area:
Buttocks region.

Benefits:
During pregnancy, the buttock muscles become strained due to the shift of weight to the front of your body. This exercise will stretch the front of the thigh, and strengthen the back of thigh and buttock muscles. This beginner buttock strengthening exercise can be performed 24 hours after giving birth.

Instruction:
Lie on back with knees bent and feet shoulder-width apart. Maintain a neutral spine position. Inhale. As you exhale, slowly pull the belly button down towards the spine. Raise buttocks off floor. Return to starting position.

Helpful Hints:
• Keep knees shoulder-width apart.
• Avoid arching back.
• Neutral spine: A position where back is not arched or flat, it is somewhere in between.

Hold:	**Repeat:**	**Frequency:**
3 – 5 seconds	2 – 10 times	2 – 3 times per day, or as tolerated.

Hip Lift with Twist

★☆☆☆☆

Target Areas:
Lower back, buttocks, and abdomen.

Benefits:
Pregnant women have a difficult time twisting their back, due to the position of the baby. This is a gentle exercise to reintroduce the body to twisting. This beginner back, buttocks, and abdominal exercise can be performed 24 hours after giving birth.

Instruction:
Lie on back with knees bent and feet shoulder-width apart. Maintain a neutral spine position. Inhale. As you exhale, slowly pull the belly button down towards the spine. Raise buttocks off floor. Slowly drop left hip toward floor while maintaining right hip level, as depicted in illustration. Keep knees steady. Raise left hip, so it is level with right hip. Repeat on opposite side.

Helpful Hints:
• Avoid arching back.
• Neutral spine: A position where back is not arched or flat, it is somewhere in between.

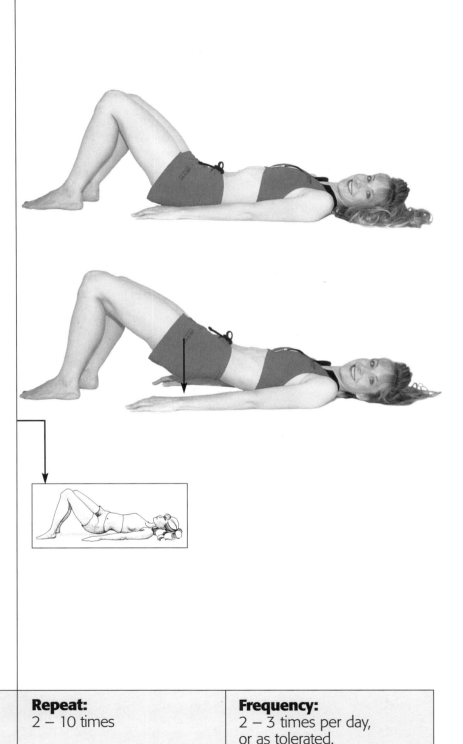

Hold:	**Repeat:**	**Frequency:**
3 - 5 seconds	2 – 10 times	2 – 3 times per day, or as tolerated.

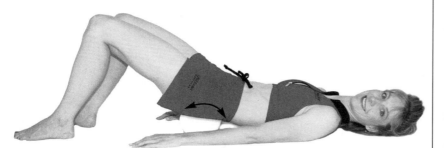

Target Areas:
Lower back and abdomen.

Benefits:
Pregnancy causes the lower back to arch, predisposing women to lower back pain. This exercise strengthens the abdomen and encourages the hips to roll back, decreasing the arch in your back. A foam roller is used with this exercise because it makes the exercise easier to do. This beginning exercise can be performed 24 hours after giving birth.

Instruction:
Lie on back with knees bent and feet shoulder-width apart. Place a half foam roller, with flat surface toward back, under your pelvis. Inhale. As you exhale, gently roll hips back flattening your spine. Return to starting position. Gently roll hips forward slightly arching spine.

Helpful Hints:
• You may also do this exercise without a foam roller.
• Do you have an exaggerated arch in your lower back while standing? If so, concentrate more on "flattening your spine".
• Avoid movement of the trunk or pelvis, and avoid using inner thigh and buttock muscles when performing exercise.
• Neutral spine: A position where back is not arched or flat, it is somewhere in between.

Hold:	**Repeat:**	**Frequency:**
3 – 5 seconds	3 – 10 times	2 – 3 times per day, or as tolerated.

Target Areas:
Abdomen and neck.

Benefits:
Diastasis recti, a separation of the long muscle in the middle of your abdomen, is common among women who have given birth. If your healthcare professional has determined that you have diastasis recti, then this exercise is for you. It will help you reduce the gap between your abdominal muscles when doing sit ups or other strenuous types of exercise.

Instruction:
Lie on your back with knees bent and feet shoulder-width apart. Place a towel or sheet underneath your back. Criss-cross towel in front of body. Grasp the towel over-handed. Inhale. Slowly pull belly button down toward spine and gently pull towel tight across your abdomen (as you exhale). Raise head off floor until *just before* you feel a gap occur in your abdomen. Keep upper back on floor.

Helpful Hint:
• To determine if you have a diastasis recti, refer to page 39.

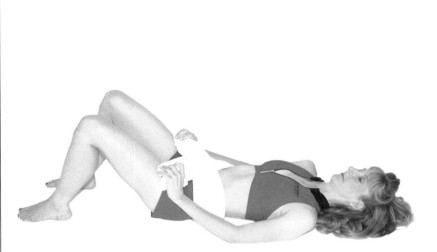

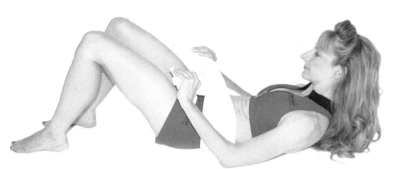

Hold:	**Repeat:**	**Frequency:**
3 seconds	2 – 10 times	2 – 3 times per day, or as tolerated.

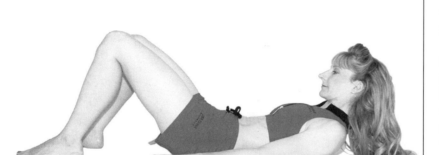

Target Areas:
Neck and abdomen.

Benefits:
Weakness of the neck and diastasis recti is common among women who have given birth. This is an excellent exercise to strengthen your neck and abdomen. When you are able to do the Assisted Neck Curl without a gap in the abdominal muscles, you may progress to this exercise.

Instruction:
Lie on your back with knees bent and feet shoulder-width apart. Slowly pull belly button down toward spine. As you exhale, raise head off floor until *just before* you feel a gap occur in your abdomen. Keep upper back on floor.

Helpful Hints:
• If you experience discomfort in your neck while performing exercise, gently place one hand behind your head for support.
• To determine if you have a diastasis recti, refer to page 39.

Hold:
3 seconds

Repeat:
2 – 10 times

Frequency:
2 – 3 times per day,
3 – 4 times per week

Neck Curl with Baby ★★☆☆☆

Target Areas:
Abdominal and neck muscles.

Benefits:
The front neck muscles become weak during pregnancy due to the change in posture. This exercise strengthens the neck muscles as well as the abdominal muscles. If you had a cesarean delivery, or have diastasis recti, begin strengthening your abdominal muscles with this exercise.

Instruction:
Lie on back with legs on ball. Place baby on abdomen. As you exhale, raise head off floor, look at baby and say GOO-CHE-GOO-CHE-GOO! Gently lower your head to floor.

Helpful Hints:
• If you have discomfort in your neck, or you feel your neck is weak, place one hand behind your head and gently raise head off floor (without pulling head forward, hand is there for support only).
• Beginners-place baby next to your side during this exercise.
• To determine if you have a diastasis recti, refer to page 39.

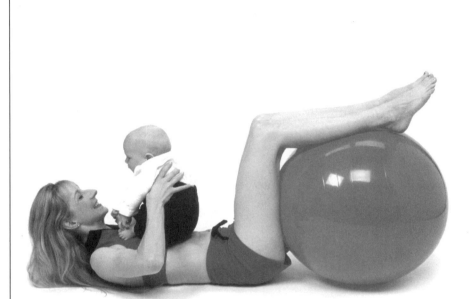

Hold:
3 seconds

Repeat: 2 sets, 3 — 12 repetitions. Rest 30 — 60 seconds between sets.

Frequency:
2 — 4 times per week

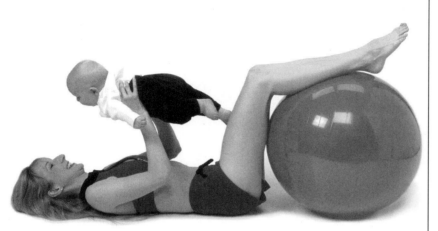

Target Areas:
Arm, chest, and shoulder muscles.

Benefits:
This exercise is an excellent way to interact with your baby socially, while strengthening your arms, chest, and shoulders. This exercise also helps baby strengthen head, trunk, and legs.

Instruction:
Lie on back with legs on ball. Hold baby on chest. Press baby up toward ceiling as you exhale. SMILE at your baby! Lower baby to chest, and kiss your baby!

Helpful Hint:
• If for any reason you feel unstable with this exercise, remove ball and place feet on ground while performing exercise.

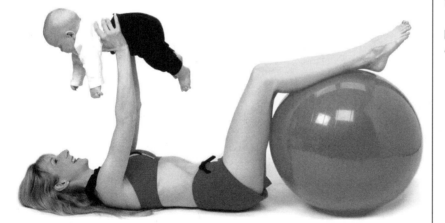

| **Hold:** 3 seconds | **Repeat:** 2 sets, 3 – 12 repetitions. Rest 30 – 60 seconds between sets. | **Frequency:** 2 – 4 times per week |

Target Areas:
Front of arms, chest, shoulder, and wrist muscles.

Benefits:
Women frequently experience weakness in their wrists and shoulders. This is an excellent beginner exercise to strengthen these areas.

Instruction:
Stand with feet shoulder-width apart. Place ball between wall and hands. Bend elbows slightly. Maintain a neutral spine by pulling belly button toward spine. Push up against ball.

Helpful Hints:
• Avoid arching back.
• Neutral spine: A position where back is not arched or flat, it is somewhere in between.

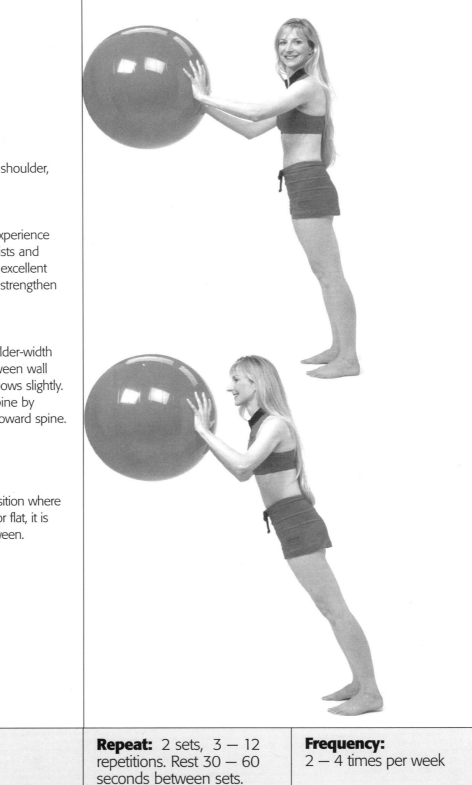

Hold:
3 seconds

Repeat: 2 sets, 3 – 12 repetitions. Rest 30 – 60 seconds between sets.

Frequency:
2 – 4 times per week

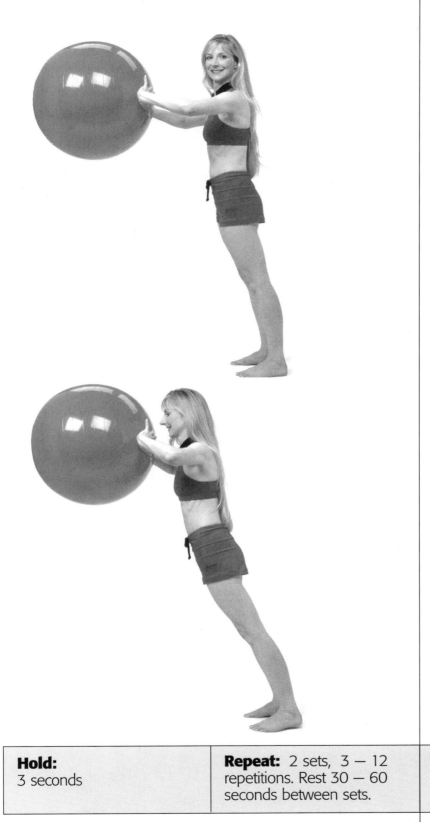

Target Areas:
Back of arms, chest, and shoulder muscles.

Benefits:
Women frequently experience drooping upper arms and weakness in their wrists and shoulders. This is an excellent toning exercise for the back of the arm droop and a good beginner exercise to strengthen the chest and shoulder muscles.

Instruction:
Stand with feet shoulder-width apart. Place ball between wall and hands. Place palm of hands on ball and turn fingers in toward each other. Bend elbows slightly. Maintain a neutral spine by pulling belly button toward spine. Push up against ball.

Helpful Hints:
- Avoid arching back by tightening abdominal muscles.
- Neutral spine: A position where back is not arched or flat, it is somewhere in between.

Hold:
3 seconds

Repeat: 2 sets, 3 — 12 repetitions. Rest 30 — 60 seconds between sets.

Frequency:
2 — 4 times per week

Target Areas:
Front of arms, chest, shoulder, and trunk muscles.

Benefits:
Pushups on a ball can be much easier or more difficult than a standard pushup. After you have mastered the wall pushup, try this advanced exercise. It will definitely challenge you.

Instruction:
Kneel. Lie with abdomen on ball. Walk arms out until ball is under thighs. Maintain a neutral spine by pulling belly button toward spine. Kiss your baby, and push up.

Helpful Hints:
• Keep back straight. Prevent abdomen from sagging by tightening abdominal muscles.
• If you have weak abdominal muscles, continue with the wall pushup until your abdominal muscles are stronger.
• To make pushup easier, roll ball closer to hands (equivalent to ★★★); to make exercise more difficult, roll ball more toward feet (equivalent to ★★★★★).
• Neutral spine: A position where back is not arched or flat, it is somewhere in between.
• Rest 30 – 60 seconds between sets of exercise.

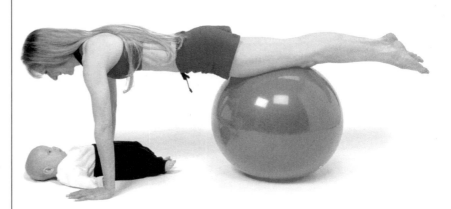

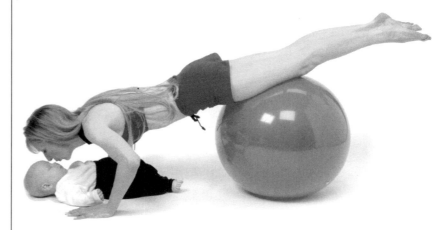

Hold:
3 seconds

Repeat:
2 sets, 5 – 15 reps.

Frequency:
2 – 4 times per week

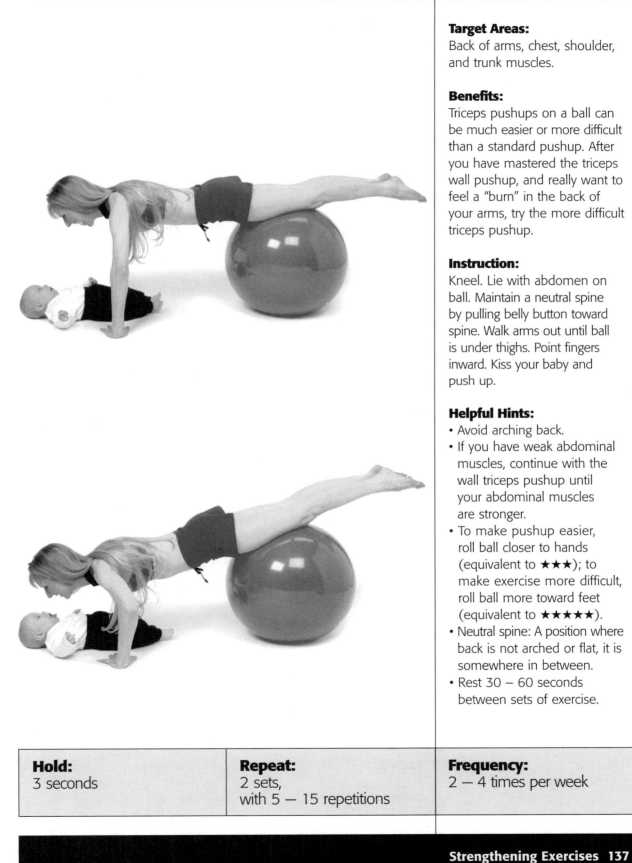

Target Areas:
Back of arms, chest, shoulder, and trunk muscles.

Benefits:
Triceps pushups on a ball can be much easier or more difficult than a standard pushup. After you have mastered the triceps wall pushup, and really want to feel a "burn" in the back of your arms, try the more difficult triceps pushup.

Instruction:
Kneel. Lie with abdomen on ball. Maintain a neutral spine by pulling belly button toward spine. Walk arms out until ball is under thighs. Point fingers inward. Kiss your baby and push up.

Helpful Hints:
• Avoid arching back.
• If you have weak abdominal muscles, continue with the wall triceps pushup until your abdominal muscles are stronger.
• To make pushup easier, roll ball closer to hands (equivalent to ★★★); to make exercise more difficult, roll ball more toward feet (equivalent to ★★★★★).
• Neutral spine: A position where back is not arched or flat, it is somewhere in between.
• Rest 30 – 60 seconds between sets of exercise.

Hold:	**Repeat:**	**Frequency:**
3 seconds	2 sets, with 5 – 15 repetitions	2 – 4 times per week

Bouncing on Ball with Baby   ★★★★☆

Target Areas:
Abdomen, buttock, thigh, trunk, and pelvic floor muscles.

Benefits:
Baby loves this exercise just as much or more than mom. The rhythmic bouncing motion helps soothe a colicky baby and assists with burping baby too. You will strengthen your abdomen, buttock, thigh, and trunk muscles, while baby works on balance, head, and trunk control. This exercise also improves urinary stress incontinence by strengthening pelvic floor muscles.

Instruction:
Sit on ball with feet shoulder-width apart. Hold baby in lap. Maintain a neutral spine by pulling belly button toward spine. To prevent urine from leaking, anticipate bouncing motions. Perform a quick flick before each bounce. Bounce up and down. Relax pelvic floor muscles prior to next bounce.

Variation:
If urinary incontinence is not an issue, perform rhythmic bouncing to soothe a fussy or colicky baby. (When urinary incontinence is not present, this exercise is equivalent to a ★.)

Helpful Hint:
• Neutral spine: A position where back is not arched or flat, it is somewhere in between.
• Avoid bouncing on ball if it causes incontinence.

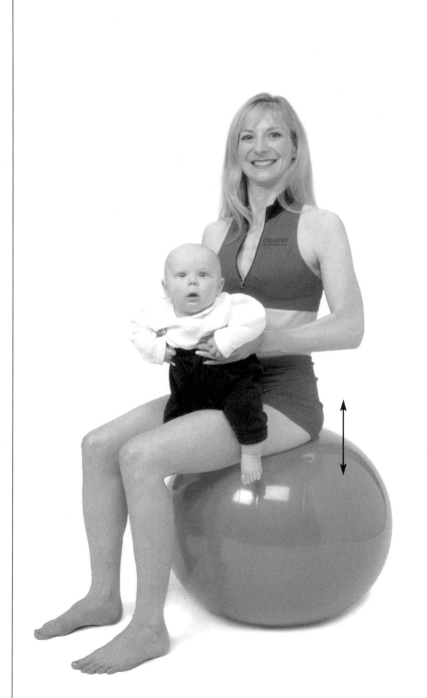

Bounce:
3 – 10 times

Repeat: 2 sets, 3 – 5 reps. Rest 60 seconds between sets

Frequency: 3 times a day, 3 – 4 times per week, OR whenever baby is fussy

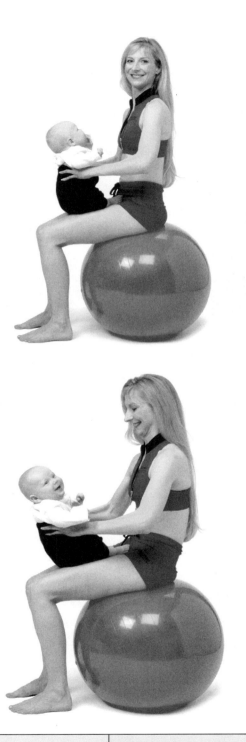

Target Area:
Abdominal muscles.

Benefits:
This exercise will strengthen lower abdominal muscles and help improve standing posture. During pregnancy, most of the additional weight gained is in the front of the body, causing the lower back to arch. This exercise helps body to reduce the "arched back" acquired during pregnancy.

Instruction:
Sit on ball with feet shoulder-width apart. Maintain a neutral spine by pulling belly button toward spine. Roll ball forward as hips roll backward (round back). Return to starting position. Roll ball backward as hips roll forward (arched back). Return to starting position.

Helpful Hints:
• Do you have an exaggerated arch in your low back in standing? If so, concentrate more on "rounding your back."
• Neutral spine: A position where back is not arched or flat, it is somewhere in between.

Hold:
3 seconds

Repeat: 2 – 3 sets, 5 – 12 reps, rest 30 – 60 seconds between sets

Frequency:
3 – 4 times per week

Target Areas:
Lower back and abdominal muscles.

Benefits:
This exercise stretches lower back muscles and strengthens lower abdominal muscles. If you have progressed from the recommended cesarean and/or diastasis recti exercises, this is a "next step" exercise appropriate for you. Baby strengthens head and back muscles.

Instruction:
Lie on back with legs on ball. Raise and place baby on top of legs. Hold onto baby's hands or arms. Pull belly button toward spine. Bend and straighten knees as far as possible without letting go of your baby.

Helpful Hint:
• To make this exercise more difficult, gently raise your head off the floor as you reach for baby and bend knees (equivalent to ★★★).

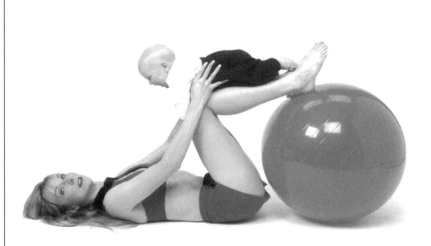

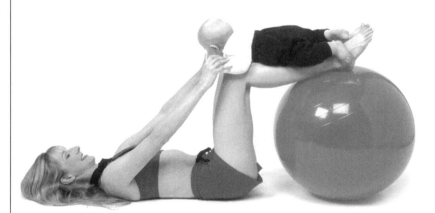

Hold: 5 seconds	**Repeat:** 2 sets, 5 — 15 reps, rest 30 — 60 seconds between sets	**Frequency:** 3 — 4 times per week

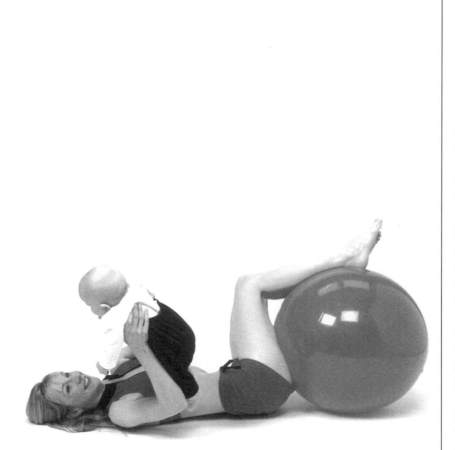

Target Areas:
Lower back and oblique abdominal (side trunk) muscles.

Benefits:
Lower back pain is common during pregnancy and after having baby. This exercise gently stretches the lower back and strengthens the oblique abdominal muscles, helping alleviate back pain.

Instruction:
Lie on back with knees bent. Place legs on ball so back of thighs touch ball. Place baby on abdomen. Pull belly button toward spine. Gently roll knees to left. To counter balance weight, gently move baby to right side of body. Maintain eye contact with baby and SMILE! Repeat in opposite direction.

Helpful Hint:
• Always try exercise without baby first (equivalent to ★★).

Hold:
5 seconds

Repeat: 2 sets, 5 — 10 reps, rest 30 — 60 seconds between sets

Frequency:
3 — 4 times per week

Target Areas:
Lower abdominal and back thigh muscles.

Benefits:
When pregnant, lower abdominal muscles s-t-r-e-t-c-h. This exercise strengthens abdominal muscles, helping to eliminate the "abdominal pooch". This exercise gives your back thigh muscles definition, too.

Instruction:
Lie on back with knees bent. Place legs on ball so back of thighs touch ball. Place baby on abdomen. Squeeze ball between heels and back of thighs. Pull belly button toward spine. Raise ball and knees toward chest as you exhale. Make eye contact with baby and enjoy this precious moment!

Helpful Hint:
• If having difficulty with this exercise, try the following: Skin contact with ball is best. Take off socks and wear shorts. Avoid lycra leggings. They make the ball slip. Or, let air out of exercise ball or use a smaller ball such as a basketball or a child's play ball.

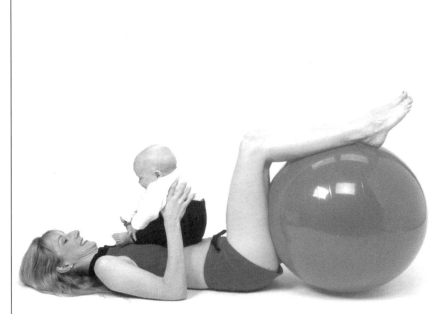

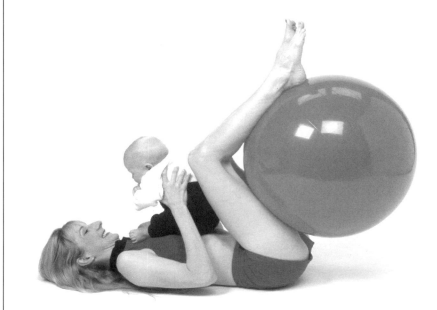

Hold:	**Repeat:** 2 sets, 5 — 15	**Frequency:**
5 seconds	reps, rest 30 — 60 seconds between sets.	2 — 4 times per week

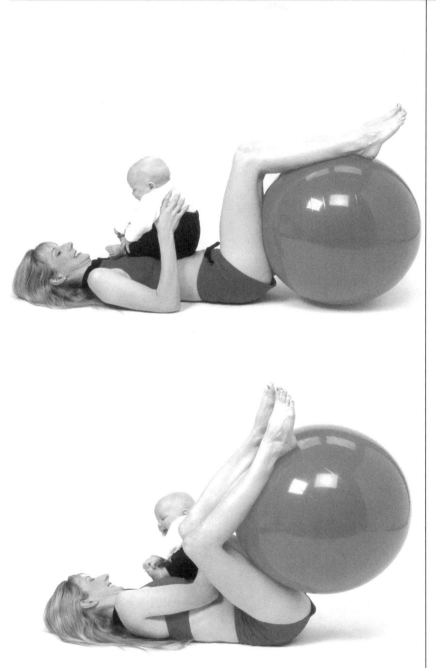

Target Area:
Oblique abdominal (side trunk) muscles.

Benefits:
Lifting the baby in and out of car seats can become very difficult, especially when baby really starts to gain weight. The oblique crunch helps strengthen side trunk muscles making it easier to lift baby out of a car seat.

Instruction:
Lie on back with knees bent. Place legs on ball so back of thighs touch ball. Place baby on abdomen. Squeeze ball between heels and back of thighs. Pull belly button toward spine. As you exhale, raise ball and knees toward left shoulder, and gently move baby to right side of body. Maintain eye contact with baby and say I LOVE YOU! Repeat in opposite direction.

Helpful Hint:
• If having difficulty with this exercise, try the following: Skin contact with ball is best. Take off socks and wear shorts. Avoid lycra leggings. They make the ball slip. Or, let air out of exercise ball or use a smaller ball such as a basketball or a child's play ball.

Hold: 5 seconds	**Repeat:** 2 sets, with 5 — 15 reps, rest 30 — 60 seconds between sets	**Frequency:** 2 — 4 times per week

Shoulder Rowing

★★☆☆☆

Target Areas:
Neck, mid-back, and shoulder muscles.

Benefits:
One of the weakest areas for many women is the mid-back region. Women who have weak mid-back muscles are more likely to slouch or exhibit poor posture. This is an excellent exercise to help promote good posture by strengthening the neck, mid-back, and shoulder muscles.

Instruction:
Kneel. Place baby on floor in front of ball. Lie with abdomen on ball. Maintain a neutral spine. Bend elbows. Raise elbows up as if rowing. Squeeze shoulder blades together. Return to starting position.

Helpful Hints:
• Avoid raising shoulders toward ears. Push shoulders down toward hips, and keep shoulders in the down position when raising elbows.
• Neutral spine: A position where back is not arched or flat, it is somewhere in between.

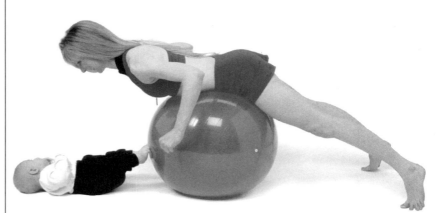

Hold:
3 seconds

Repeat: 2 sets, with 5 — 12 reps, rest 30 — 60 seconds between sets

Frequency:
3 — 4 times per week

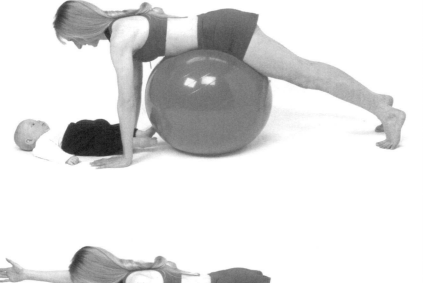

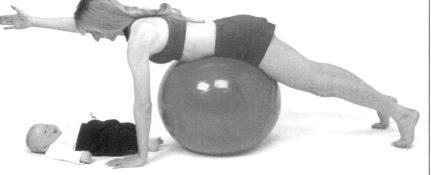

Target Areas:
Arm, mid-back, and neck muscles.

Benefits:
Women who have weak mid-back muscles are more likely to slouch or exhibit poor posture. This is an excellent exercise to help promote good posture by strengthening the neck, mid-back, and shoulder muscles.

Instruction:
Kneel. Place baby on floor in front of ball. Lie with abdomen on ball. Maintain a neutral spine by pulling belly button toward spine. Raise one hand, with thumb up, to ear height. Repeat with opposite hand.

Helpful Hints:
• Relax shoulders when doing exercise.
• Neutral spine: A position where back is not arched or flat, it is somewhere in between.

Hold:	**Repeat:** 2 sets, with	**Frequency:**
3 seconds	5 — 12 reps, rest 30 — 60 seconds between sets	3 — 4 times per week

Back Strengthener with Leg Raise

★★☆☆☆

Target Areas:
Back, buttock, neck, and back of thigh muscles.

Benefits:
Lower back pain is common during pregnancy and after baby is born. This exercise will help prevent or alleviate lower back pain by strengthening the lower back and surrounding muscles.

Instruction:
Kneel. Place baby on floor in front of ball. Lie with abdomen on ball. Maintain neutral spine by pulling belly button toward spine. Raise left heel to buttock height. Repeat with opposite leg.

Helpful Hints:
• Avoid lifting leg so high that back rotates.
• Neutral spine: A position where back is not arched or flat, it is somewhere in between.

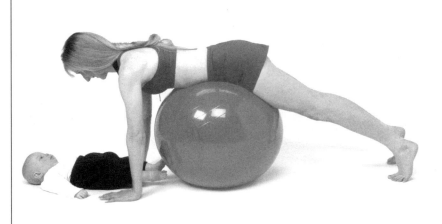

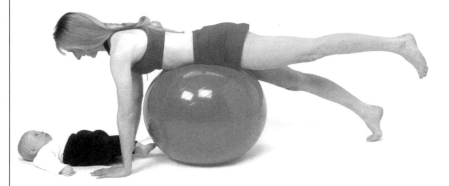

Hold: 3 seconds	**Repeat:** 2 sets, with 5 — 12 reps, rest 30 seconds between sets	**Frequency:** 3 — 4 times per week

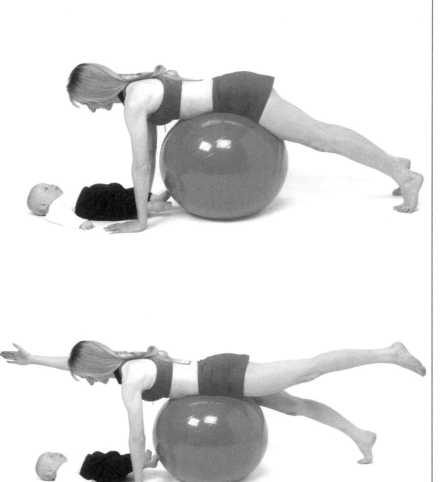

Target Areas:
Arm, back, buttock, neck, and back of thigh muscles.

Benefits:
Poor posture and lower back pain are common during pregnancy and after baby is born. This exercise will help prevent or alleviate lower back pain by strengthening the lower back and surrounding muscles. It encourages upper and lower body muscles to work together.

Instruction:
Kneel. Place baby on floor in front of ball. Lie with abdomen on ball. Maintain a neutral spine by pulling belly button toward spine. Raise left heel to buttock height and right hand, with thumb up, to ear height. Repeat with opposite arm and leg.

Helpful Hints:
• Avoid lifting leg or hand so high that back rotates.
• Neutral spine: A position where back is not arched or flat, it is somewhere in between.

Hold: 3 seconds	**Repeat:** 2 sets, 5 — 12 reps, rest 30 — 60 seconds between sets	**Frequency:** 3 — 4 times per week

Target Area:
Back muscles.

Benefits:
This exercise is for beginners and is great for strengthening the lower back of a new mother. Strengthening your back will make it easier to lift your baby in and out of a high chair.

Instruction:
Place baby on floor and ball next to baby's feet. Kneel. Lie with abdomen on ball and upper body over top of ball. Cross arms in front of body. Maintain a neutral spine by pulling belly button toward spine. Raise chest up. Return to starting position.

Helpful Hints:
• Keep back straight, and avoid arching back.
• If feet slip on floor, place feet against wall or other solid object.
• Neutral spine: A position where back is not arched or flat, it is somewhere in between.

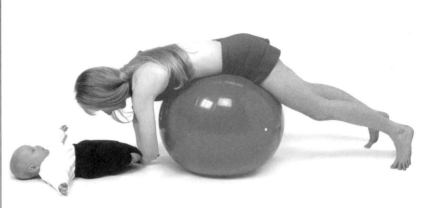

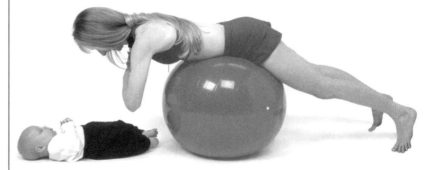

Hold:
5 seconds

Repeat: 2 sets,
3 — 12 reps, rest 30 – 60 seconds between sets

Frequency:
3 — 4 times per week

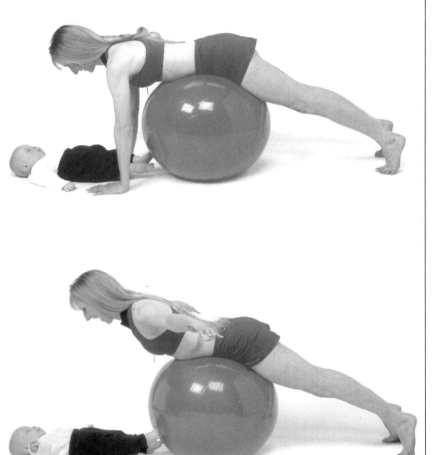

Target Areas:
Arm, back, and neck muscles.

Benefits:
This intermediate exercise is great for strengthening the mid and lower back of a new mother.

Instruction:
Kneel. Place baby on floor in front of ball. Lie with abdomen on ball. Extend legs. Maintain a neutral spine by pulling belly button toward spine. Raise chest off ball as hands are raised out to side of body with palms down. Watch your baby mimic your movements! Return to starting position.

Helpful Hints:
• If feet slide with exercise or you have a difficult time lifting chest off ball, place feet against wall for stability.
• Neutral spine: A position where back is not arched or flat, it is somewhere in between.

Hold:
3 – 5 seconds

Repeat: 2 sets, with 3 – 12 reps, rest 30 – 60 seconds between sets

Frequency:
2 – 4 times per week

Superwoman ★★★★★

Target Areas:
Arm, back, and neck muscles.

Benefits:
Poor posture and lower back pain are common during pregnancy and after baby is born. This advanced exercise will help prevent or alleviate lower back pain by strengthening the entire back. It encourages upper and lower body muscles to work together.

Instruction:
Kneel. Place baby on floor in front of ball. Lie with abdomen on ball. Extend legs. Maintain a neutral spine by pulling belly button toward spine. Raise chest off ball as hands are raised overhead with thumbs up. Return to starting position.

Helpful Hints:
• Keep back straight, and avoid arching back.
• If feet slide with exercise or you have a difficult time lifting chest off ball, place feet against wall for stability.
• Neutral spine: A position where back is not arched or flat, it is somewhere in between.

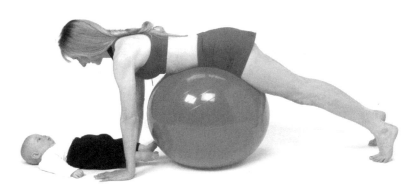
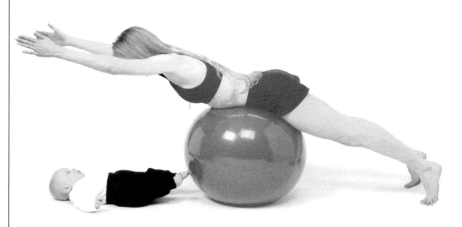

Hold:
3 – 5 seconds

Repeat: 2 sets, with 3 – 12 reps, rest 30 – 60 seconds between sets

Frequency:
2 – 4 times per week

150 Strengthening Exercises

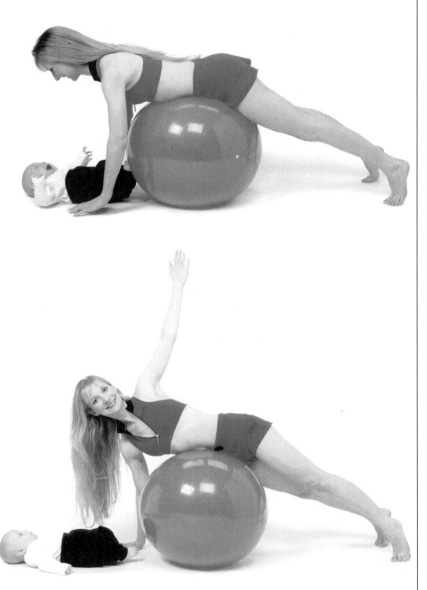

Target Areas:
Abdominal and back muscles.

Benefits:
As your pregnancy progresses, it becomes more and more difficult to rotate the torso. After the baby is born, it is very important to strengthen the abdominal and back muscles that assist with trunk rotation. This exercise will help improve trunk range of motion and strength.

Instruction:
Kneel. Place baby on floor in front of ball. Lie with abdomen on ball, and pull belly button toward spine. Lift left arm out to side of body. Rotate torso as arm is raised to ceiling. Follow hand motion with eyes. Keep hips on ball. Return to starting position. Repeat with opposite side.

Helpful Hint:
• Avoid lifting hips and/or pelvis off ball.

Hold:	**Repeat:** 2 sets,	**Frequency:**
3 seconds	5 — 12 reps, rest 30 — 60 seconds between sets	3 — 4 times per week

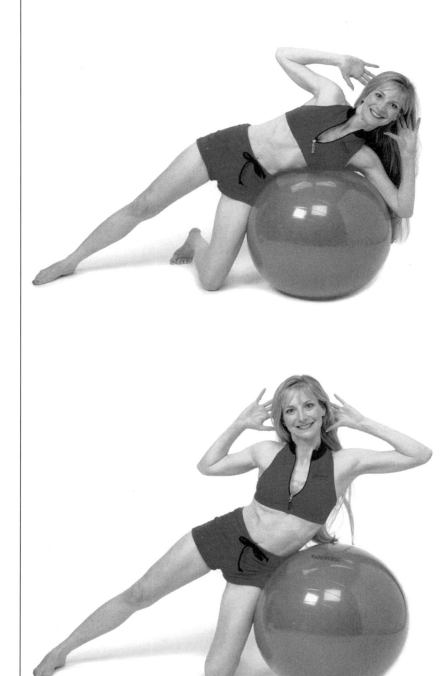

Target Area:
Side abdominal muscles.

Benefits:
As your pregnancy progresses, it becomes more and more difficult to bend your torso sideways. After the baby is born, it is very important to strengthen the abdominal muscles that assist with trunk side bending, as this exercise does.

Instruction:
Kneel. Place ball alongside body. Straighten top leg and place unclasped hands behind head. Pull belly button toward spine. Side bend body while raising trunk off ball. Repeat with opposite side.

Helpful Hints:
• Keep a straight line between ankle, hips, and shoulders when raising trunk off ball. If you are unable to keep a straight line when lifting off ball, try raising trunk only 4 inches off ball.
• If you're having difficulty keeping your balance, place top foot against wall.

Hold:
3 seconds

Repeat: 2 sets, with 3 — 12 reps, rest 60 seconds between sets

Frequency:
2 — 4 times per week

Target Areas:
Outer thigh and hip muscles.

Benefits:
When holding baby on hip, (right handed women tend to hold baby on left hip) we tend to hike up and push out the hip (see photo page 71) to provide a small ledge for the baby to rest upon. This motion stretches the hip and thigh muscles causing weakness in these areas. This exercise will help strengthen the outer thigh and hip muscles.

Instruction:
Kneel. Hold baby in front of ball. Place ball alongside body. Straighten top leg. Maintain a neutral spine by pulling belly button toward spine. Raise top leg with foot parallel to floor to hip height.

Helpful Hints:
• Keep a straight line between ankle, hips, and shoulders. (Most exercises tend to bring the ankle in front of hip, this makes the exercise easier but strengthens a different muscle).
• If you are able to raise ankle higher than hip, you are probably doing exercise incorrectly.
• Neutral spine: A position where back is not arched or flat, it is somewhere in between.
• If you're having difficulty keeping your balance, place baby on floor, and/or place ball against wall (equivalent to ★★).

Hold:
3 seconds

Repeat: 2 sets, with 5 — 12 reps, rest 30 — 60 seconds between sets

Frequency:
3 — 4 times per week

Target Areas:
Inner thigh and pelvic
floor muscles.

Benefits:
Strengthens and tones inner thigh
and pelvic floor muscles. Squeezing
the ball may also relieve pain in
pubic bone region by helping to
align the pubic bones.

Instruction:
Lie on side with ball between
ankles. Straighten legs. Place
baby in front of body. Squeeze
ankles together and draw pelvic
floor muscles up and in, as with
a Kegel exercise. Relax.

Helpful Hints:
• Keep a straight line between
  ankle, hips, and shoulders.
  (Most people tend to bring the
  ankle in front of hip, making
  exercise easier but strengthening
  a different muscle.)
• Alternate baby position: Place
  baby on floor along your side.

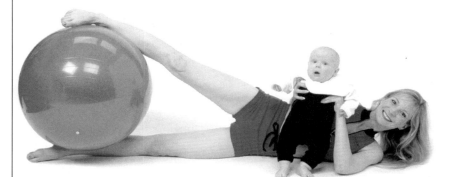

Hold:
3 seconds

Repeat: 2 sets, with
5 – 12 reps, rest 30 – 60
seconds between sets

Frequency:
3 – 4 times per week

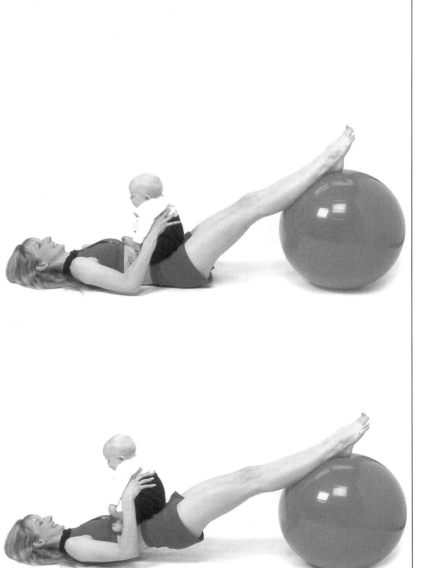

Target Areas:
Buttock and back of thigh muscles.

Benefits:
This exercise will strengthen legs, making stair climbing with baby much easier.

Instruction:
Lie on back. Place feet on ball and baby on abdomen. Maintain a neutral spine by pulling belly button toward spine. Keeping legs straight, lift hips off floor. Return to starting position.

Helpful Hints:
• Always try exercises without baby first. When you become proficient with this exercise, you may begin exercising with baby.
• Avoid arching back.
• This is an excellent position to strengthen pelvic floor muscles by performing a Kegel, since gravity will assist your muscles.
• Neutral spine: A position where back is not arched or flat, it is somewhere in between.

Hold:	**Repeat:** 2 sets, with	**Frequency:**
5 seconds	5 — 15 reps, rest 30 — 60 seconds between sets	2 — 4 times per week

Target Areas:
Lower back, buttock and back of thigh muscles.

Benefits:
This exercise will strengthen legs, making stroller pushing up hill much easier.

Instruction:
Lie on back. Place feet on ball and baby on abdomen. Maintain a neutral spine by pulling belly button toward spine. Bend knees and lift hips off floor. Return to starting position.

Helpful Hints:
• Always try exercises without baby first. When you become proficient with the exercise, you may begin exercising with baby.
• Avoid arching back.
• Neutral spine: A position where back is not arched or flat, it is somewhere in between.

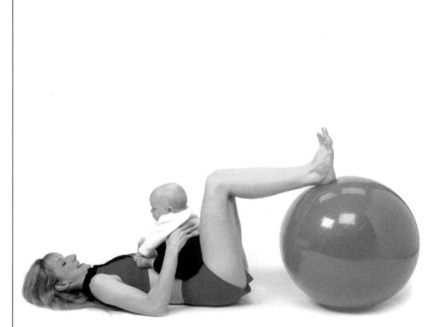

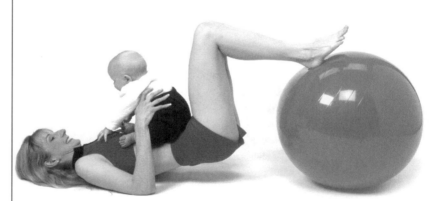

Hold:
5 seconds

Repeat: 2 sets, with 5 — 15 reps, rest 30 — 60 seconds between sets

Frequency:
2 — 4 times per week

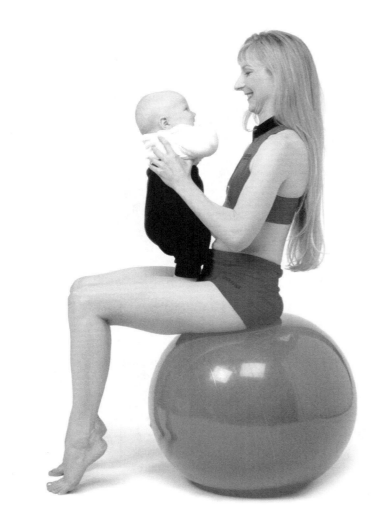

Target Area:
Small calf muscles.

Benefits:
Strengthens calf muscles, preparing mom for rocking baby to sleep.

Instruction:
Sit on ball with feet shoulder-width apart. Hold baby in lap. Maintain a neutral position by pulling belly button toward spine. Raise heels off floor. Return to starting position.

Helpful Hints:
• Alternate exercise: Follow directions as above, however, raise and lower heels as fast as you can.
• Neutral spine: A position where back is not arched or flat, it is somewhere in between.

Hold:
3 seconds

Repeat: 2 sets, with 12 reps, rest 30 seconds between sets

Frequency:
2 — 4 times per week

Target Area:
Shin muscles.

Benefits:
Strengthens shin muscles, preparing mom for rocking baby to sleep. Strong shin muscles prevent "shin splints" from occurring.

Instruction:
Sit on ball with feet shoulder-width apart. Maintain a neutral position by pulling belly button toward spine. Hold baby in lap. Raise toes off floor.

Helpful Hints:
• Alternate exercise: Follow directions as above, however tap toes on floor as fast as you can.
• Neutral spine: A position where back is not arched or flat, it is somewhere in between.

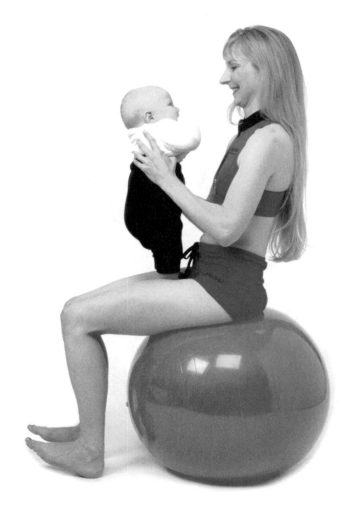

Hold:
3 seconds

Repeat:
2 sets, with 12 reps, rest 30 seconds between sets

Frequency:
2 — 4 times per week

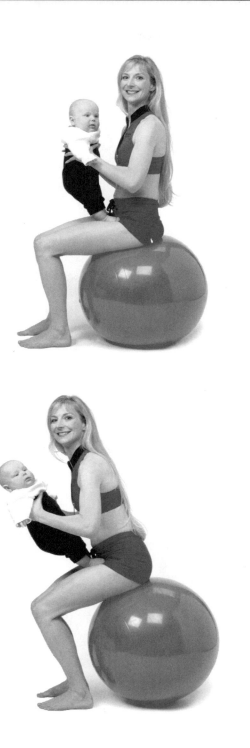

Target Areas:
Buttock and thigh muscles.

Benefits:
Strengthens legs and buttock muscles, making it easier for mom to go from a sitting position to a standing position while holding baby. This exercise also helps strengthen pelvic floor muscles preventing urinary stress incontinence.

Instruction:
Sit on ball with feet shoulder-width apart. Maintain a neutral back by pulling belly button toward spine. Hold baby on lap. Quickly flick pelvic floor muscles up and in while slowly leaning forward. Body weight should be evenly distributed and knees aligned over feet. Return to starting position.

Helpful Hints:
• To prevent ball from rolling away, avoid raising buttocks off ball.
• If you would like an additional "thigh burner" exercise, follow directions as above holding for 30 – 60 seconds.
• Neutral spine: A position where back is not arched or flat, it is somewhere in between.

Hold:
3 – 5 seconds

Repeat: 2 sets, with 5 – 12 reps, rest 30 – 60 seconds between sets

Frequency:
3 – 4 times per week

Target Areas:
Thigh and calf muscles.

Benefits:
This exercise will strengthen your calf and thigh muscles, better preparing you for lifting your growing baby.

Instruction:
Sit on ball with baby in lap. Rotate body to right, resting baby gently on right thigh, and extend left leg backward. Keep feet and knees aligned. Maintain a neutral spine by pulling belly button toward spine. Return to starting position. Repeat on opposite side.

Helpful Hints:
• Avoid arching back.
• Neutral spine: A position where back is not arched or flat, it is somewhere in between.

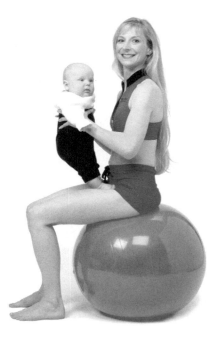

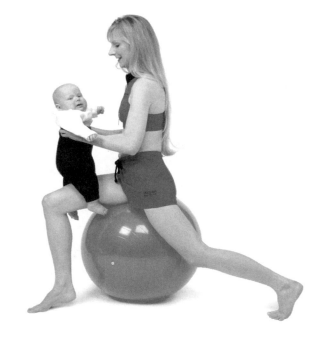

Hold:
5 seconds

Repeat: 2 sets, 5 — 12 reps, rest 60 seconds between sets

Frequency:
2 — 4 times per week

Target Areas:
Buttock and thigh muscles.

Benefits:
Prepares leg and buttock muscles for proper lifting of baby.

Instruction:
Stand with feet shoulder-width apart. Place ball between small curve in back and wall. Hold baby in front of body. Maintain a neutral spine by pulling belly button toward spine. Bend knees. Smile at your baby!

Helpful Hints:
• Beginners, do this exercise without your baby until your legs are stronger.
• If you would like an additional "thigh burner" exercise, follow directions as above holding for 30 — 60 seconds.
• Alternate Baby Position: Hug your baby close to your body. This will place less stress on your abdomen, arms and back.
• Neutral spine: A position where back is not arched or flat, it is somewhere in between.

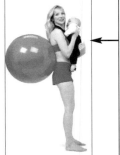

Hold:
3 seconds

Repeat: 2 sets, 5 — 12 reps, rest 30 seconds between sets

Frequency:
3 — 4 times per week

Target Areas:
Abdominal, back, calf, thigh, and pelvic floor muscles.

Benefits:
This exercise strengthens your abdomen, back, calf, thigh, and pelvic floor muscles. It also teaches your body how to coordinate a pelvic floor contraction with other muscles. This is extremely important in lifting, running, jumping, or playing with your baby.

Instruction:
Stand with feet shoulder-width apart. Place ball between small curve in back and wall. Hug or hold baby in front of body. Maintain a neutral spine by pulling belly button toward spine. Bend knees and raise heels off floor. Press up into a standing position while pulling pelvic floor muscles up and in (as with a Kegel exercise). Relax and return to standing position.

Helpful Hints:
• *Begin exercise without baby.*
  The weight of the baby will make it difficult to contract/tighten pelvic floor muscles. When you add your baby to the exercise, begin with the baby hug position as demonstrated.
• Neutral spine: A position where back is not arched or flat, it is somewhere in between.

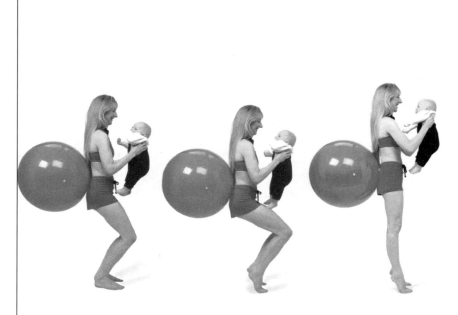

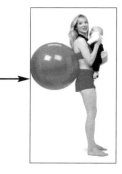

Hold:
3 seconds

Repeat: 2 sets, 5 — 12 reps, rest 60 seconds between sets

Frequency:
2 — 4 times per week

FLOW CHART

Date: Exercise:	Set	Hold Time	1	2	3	Exercise Heart Rate	Hold Time	1	2	3	Exercise Heart Rate	Hold Time	1	2	3	Exercise Heart Rate	Hold Time	1	2	3	Exercise Heart Rate
Chest and finger Stretch	**Rep**	20	3	–	–	100															
Transverse Abdominis	**Rep**	5	5	5	–	–															
Airplane	**Rep**	–	8	8	–	140															
	Rep																				
	Rep																				
	Rep																				
	Rep																				
	Rep																				
	Rep																				
	Rep																				
	Rep																				
	Rep																				
	Rep																				
	Rep																				
	Rep																				
	Rep																				
	Rep																				
	Rep																				
	Rep																				
	Rep																				
	Rep																				
	Rep																				
	Rep																				
	Rep																				
	Rep																				
	Rep																				
	Rep																				
	Rep																				
	Rep																				

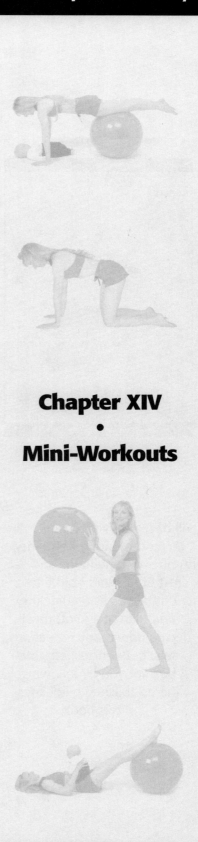

Chapter XIV
•
Mini-Workouts

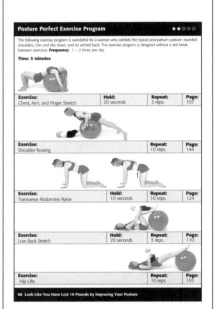

14.1 Posture Perfect Exercise Program

All of the mini-workouts have a recommended frequency, number of repetitions and sets, rest break, and hold times. This serves as a guideline, and ultimately, you must decide how many repetitions, sets, frequencies, etc., are best for you by following the established guidelines in this book.

Mini-Workouts

The mini-workouts are designed as a quick reference to the exercises illustrated throughout the book, and to give you workout routine ideas (see illustration 14.1). Perform these routines only after reading this entire book and then performing the exercises as illustrated on the specified pages.

I designed the *Bouncing Back Into Shape After Baby* mini-workouts to provide time-efficient workouts that can be squeezed into any part of your day. Each workout takes 10 minutes, or less, to perform. These mini-workouts may be used one at a time or several at a time to make a 20 or 30-minute workout.

Each of the mini-workouts has been rated on a one to five star system. One star signifies the most basic exercise level, two stars – advanced beginner, three stars – intermediate, four stars – advanced, and five stars – expert. The star rating is located at the top of the page. If the workout received one star, then you will know right away that this workout may be performed by a beginner, and a five star workout means you may need to wait awhile before you perform this exercise, or that this exercise is for you if you are already in great shape.

Once you have mastered all the one – star workouts, progress to two – star workouts. Progress to the next level of difficulty only after perfecting your current workout level. Keep in mind, it is more difficult to perform a workout routine than it is to perform individual exercises. Five one-star exercises performed consecutively is much more difficult than performing a single one star exercise.

All of the mini-workouts have a recommended frequency, number of repetitions and sets, rest break, and hold times. This serves as a guideline, and ultimately, you must decide how many repetitions, sets, frequencies, etc., are best for you by following the established guidelines in this book.

I hope you enjoy these fun, time and energy-efficient workouts. The mini-workout pages are perforated so you may tear them out, post them on a wall, or take them with you.

The following exercise progression is appropriate for women within 24 hours after vaginal delivery, with physician's or physical therapist's consent. These exercises are also appropriate for a woman with diastasis recti. **Rest** between exercises as needed. **Frequency:** Perform 2 – 3 times per day or as tolerated. **Time: 5 minutes + 5 minute walk**

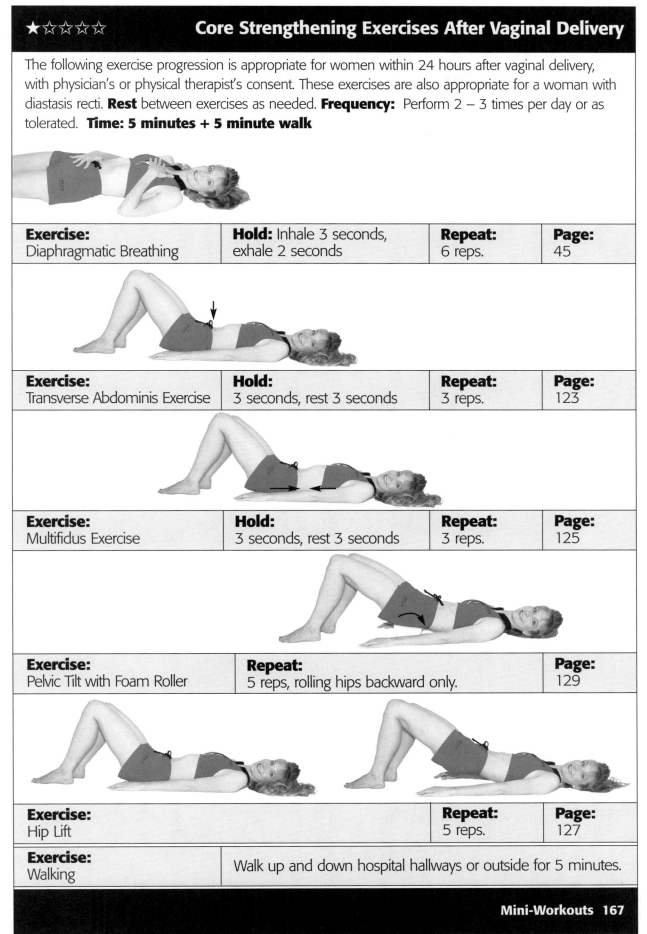

Exercise: Diaphragmatic Breathing	**Hold:** Inhale 3 seconds, exhale 2 seconds	**Repeat:** 6 reps.	**Page:** 45

Exercise: Transverse Abdominis Exercise	**Hold:** 3 seconds, rest 3 seconds	**Repeat:** 3 reps.	**Page:** 123

Exercise: Multifidus Exercise	**Hold:** 3 seconds, rest 3 seconds	**Repeat:** 3 reps.	**Page:** 125

Exercise: Pelvic Tilt with Foam Roller	**Repeat:** 5 reps, rolling hips backward only.	**Page:** 129

Exercise: Hip Lift	**Repeat:** 5 reps.	**Page:** 127

Exercise: Walking	Walk up and down hospital hallways or outside for 5 minutes.

Core Strengthening Exercises After Cesarean Delivery ★☆☆☆☆

The following exercise progression is appropriate for women within 24 hours after cesarean delivery, with physician's or physical therapist's consent. These exercises are also appropriate for a woman with diastasis recti. **Rest** between exercises as needed. **Frequency:** Perform 2 – 3 times per day or as tolerated. **Time: 5 minutes + 5 minute walk**

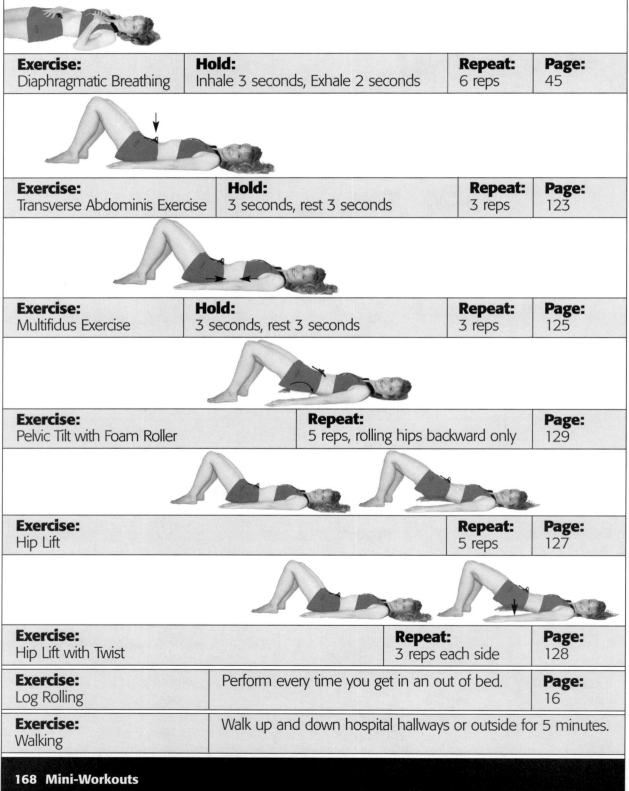

Exercise: Diaphragmatic Breathing	**Hold:** Inhale 3 seconds, Exhale 2 seconds		**Repeat:** 6 reps	**Page:** 45
Exercise: Transverse Abdominis Exercise	**Hold:** 3 seconds, rest 3 seconds		**Repeat:** 3 reps	**Page:** 123
Exercise: Multifidus Exercise	**Hold:** 3 seconds, rest 3 seconds		**Repeat:** 3 reps	**Page:** 125
Exercise: Pelvic Tilt with Foam Roller		**Repeat:** 5 reps, rolling hips backward only		**Page:** 129
Exercise: Hip Lift			**Repeat:** 5 reps	**Page:** 127
Exercise: Hip Lift with Twist		**Repeat:** 3 reps each side		**Page:** 128
Exercise: Log Rolling	Perform every time you get in an out of bed.			**Page:** 16
Exercise: Walking	Walk up and down hospital hallways or outside for 5 minutes.			

The following exercise progression is appropriate for a woman with diastasis recti. Progress to exercise number 5, Neck Curl, when you are able to do a Neck Curl without having a bulge, or diastasis recti. **Rest:** between exercises as needed. **Frequency:** Perform 2 – 3 times per day as tolerated. **Time: 5 minutes**

Exercise:	Repeat:	Page:
Transverse Abdominis Exercise	10 reps 5 –10 seconds	123

Exercise:	Repeat:	Page:
Multifidus Exercise	10 reps, 5 –10 seconds	125

Exercise:	Repeat:	Page:
Neck Curl Assisted	2 –10 reps, 3 seconds	130

Exercise:	Repeat:	Page:
Pelvic Tilt with Foam Roller	10 reps, rolling hips backward only	129

Exercise:	Repeat:	Page:
Neck Curl	10 reps	131

Core Strengthening Abdominal Exercise Progression ★★☆☆☆

Master this exercise regimen before progressing on to ★★★ or ★★★★ mini-workouts. These exercises are also appropriate for a woman with diastasis recti. **Rest:** 30 seconds between exercises or as needed. **Frequency:** Perform 1 – 3 times per day or as tolerated. **Time: 10 minutes**

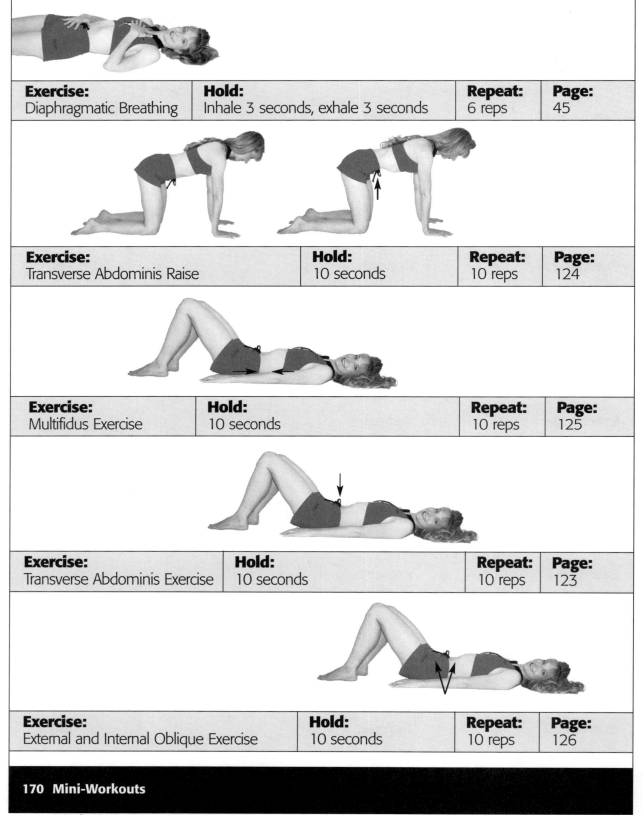

Exercise:	Hold:	Repeat:	Page:
Diaphragmatic Breathing	Inhale 3 seconds, exhale 3 seconds	6 reps	45

Exercise:	Hold:	Repeat:	Page:
Transverse Abdominis Raise	10 seconds	10 reps	124

Exercise:	Hold:	Repeat:	Page:
Multifidus Exercise	10 seconds	10 reps	125

Exercise:	Hold:	Repeat:	Page:
Transverse Abdominis Exercise	10 seconds	10 reps	123

Exercise:	Hold:	Repeat:	Page:
External and Internal Oblique Exercise	10 seconds	10 reps	126

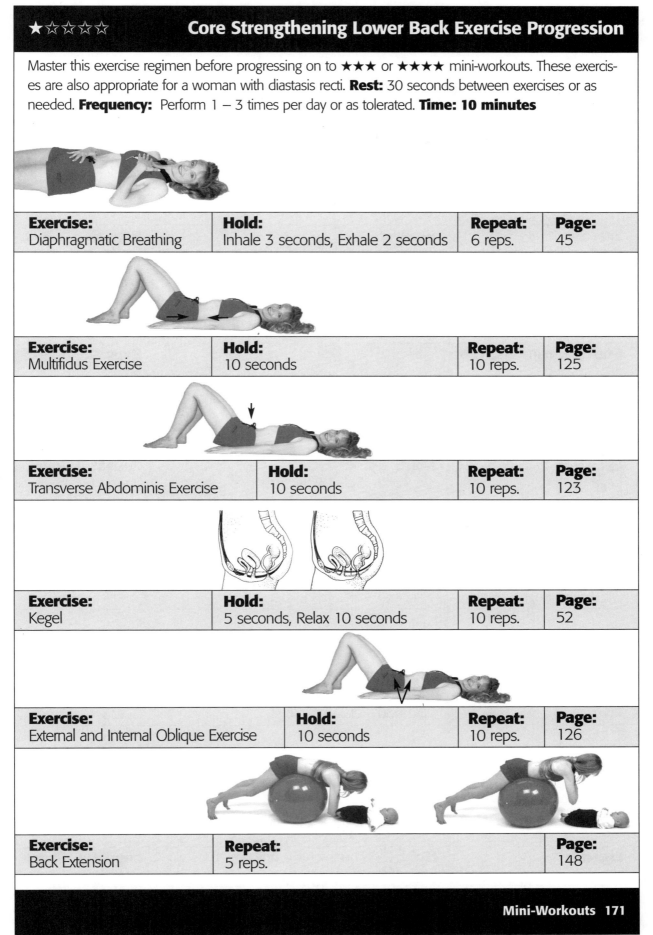

Core Strengthening Lower Back Exercise Progression

★☆☆☆☆

Master this exercise regimen before progressing on to ★★★ or ★★★★ mini-workouts. These exercises are also appropriate for a woman with diastasis recti. **Rest:** 30 seconds between exercises or as needed. **Frequency:** Perform 1 – 3 times per day or as tolerated. **Time: 10 minutes**

Exercise: Diaphragmatic Breathing	Hold: Inhale 3 seconds, Exhale 2 seconds	Repeat: 6 reps.	Page: 45

Exercise: Multifidus Exercise	Hold: 10 seconds	Repeat: 10 reps.	Page: 125

Exercise: Transverse Abdominis Exercise	Hold: 10 seconds	Repeat: 10 reps.	Page: 123

Exercise: Kegel	Hold: 5 seconds, Relax 10 seconds	Repeat: 10 reps.	Page: 52

Exercise: External and Internal Oblique Exercise	Hold: 10 seconds	Repeat: 10 reps.	Page: 126

Exercise: Back Extension	Repeat: 5 reps.		Page: 148

Basic Pelvic Floor Exercise Progression   ★☆☆☆☆

Performing a pelvic floor exercise workout is more difficult than doing the exercises individually. Master individual exercises before performing this mini-workout. Perfect this exercise regimen before progressing on to ★★★ or ★★★★★ mini-workouts. **Rest:** 60 seconds between exercises or as needed. **Frequency:** Perform 1- 3 times per day or as tolerated.

Time: 10 minutes

Exercise:	Hold:	Repeat:	Page:
Exercise: Diaphragmatic Breathing	**Hold:** Inhale 3 seconds, Exhale 2 seconds	**Repeat:** 6 reps.	**Page:** 45

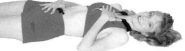

Exercise: Transverse Abdominis Raise with Kegel Ball Squeeze	**Hold:** 3 seconds, Relax 6 seconds	**Repeat:** 5 reps.	**Page:** 51
Exercise: Kegel	**Hold:** 3 seconds, Relax 6 seconds	**Repeat:** 5 reps.	**Page:** 52
Exercise: Quick Flick Kegel	**Hold:** 1 second, Relax completely	**Repeat:** 5 reps.	**Page:** 56
Exercise: Tail Wagging	**Hold:** 1 second, Relax completely	**Repeat:** 5 reps.	**Page:** 57
Exercise: Advanced Kegel	**Hold:** 5 seconds while breathing in Relax: 5 seconds while breathing out	**Repeat:** 3 reps.	**Page:** 53
Exercise: Elevator Exercise	**Hold:** 2 seconds on each floor Relax: 8 seconds	**Repeat:** 3 reps.	**Page:** 54

The following exercise program is wonderful for a woman who exhibits the typical postpartum posture: rounded shoulders, chin and ribs down, and an arched back. This exercise program is designed without a rest break between exercises. **Frequency:** 1 – 2 times per day.

Time: 5 minutes

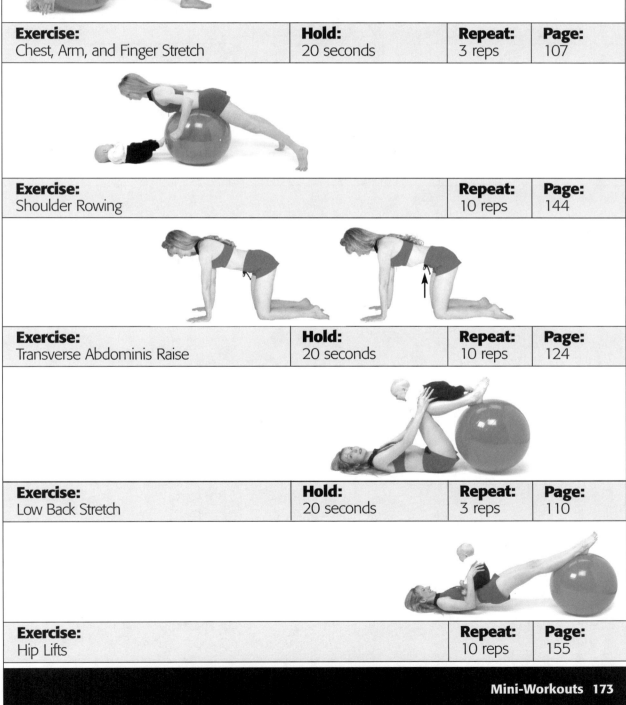

Exercise: Chest, Arm, and Finger Stretch	**Hold:** 20 seconds	**Repeat:** 3 reps	**Page:** 107

Exercise: Shoulder Rowing		**Repeat:** 10 reps	**Page:** 144

Exercise: Transverse Abdominis Raise	**Hold:** 20 seconds	**Repeat:** 10 reps	**Page:** 124

Exercise: Low Back Stretch	**Hold:** 20 seconds	**Repeat:** 3 reps	**Page:** 110

Exercise: Hip Lifts		**Repeat:** 10 reps	**Page:** 155

★ ☆ ☆ ☆ ☆

The following stretching program can be used before or after an aerobic or strengthening workout, or any time throughout the day. This exercise program is designed without a rest break between stretches. **Frequency:** 1 – 2 times per day. **Time: 8 minutes**

Exercise: Side Neck Stretch	**Hold:** 20 seconds	**Repeat:** 2 reps each side	**Page:** 100

Exercise: Back of Neck Stretch	**Hold:** 20 seconds	**Repeat:** 2 reps each side	**Page:** 101

Exercise: Back of Wrist Stretch	**Hold:** 20 seconds	**Repeat:** 2 reps	**Page:** 103

Exercise: Front of Wrist Stretch	**Hold:** 20 seconds	**Repeat:** 2 reps	**Page:** 102

Exercise: Shoulder Roll Stretch	**Hold:** 20 seconds	**Repeat:** 2 reps each side	**Page:** 105

Exercise: Nerve Stretch	**Hold:** 20 seconds	**Repeat:** 2 reps each side	**Page:** 106

The following stretching program can be used before or after an aerobic or strengthening workout, or any time throughout the day. This exercise program is designed without a rest break between stretches. **Frequency:** 1 – 2 times per day. **Time: 6 minutes**

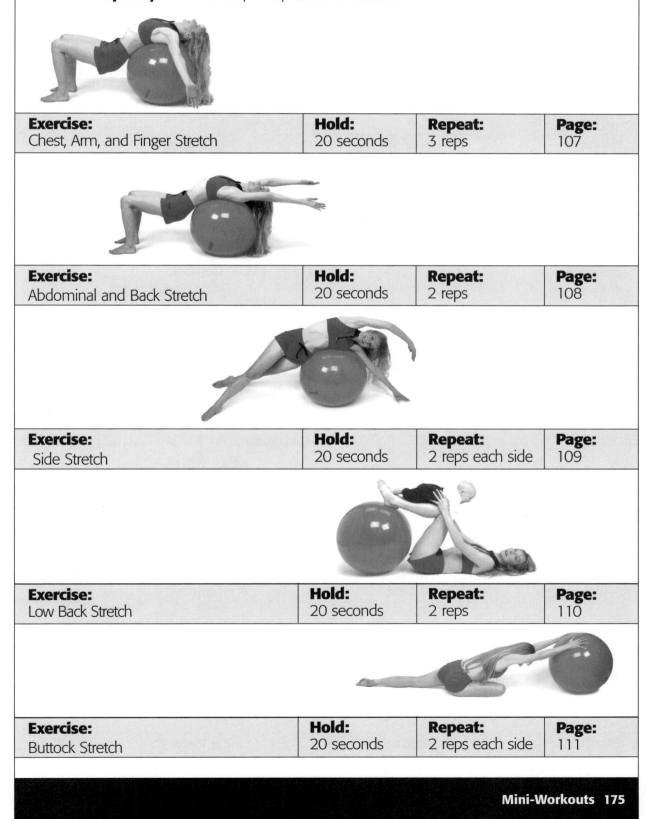

Exercise:	Hold:	Repeat:	Page:
Chest, Arm, and Finger Stretch	20 seconds	3 reps	107

Exercise:	Hold:	Repeat:	Page:
Abdominal and Back Stretch	20 seconds	2 reps	108

Exercise:	Hold:	Repeat:	Page:
Side Stretch	20 seconds	2 reps each side	109

Exercise:	Hold:	Repeat:	Page:
Low Back Stretch	20 seconds	2 reps	110

Exercise:	Hold:	Repeat:	Page:
Buttock Stretch	20 seconds	2 reps each side	111

Lower Body Stretches ★☆☆☆☆

The following stretching program can be used before or after an aerobic or strengthening workout, or any time throughout the day. This exercise program is designed without a rest break between stretches.

Frequency: 1 – 2 times per day. **Time: 10 minutes**

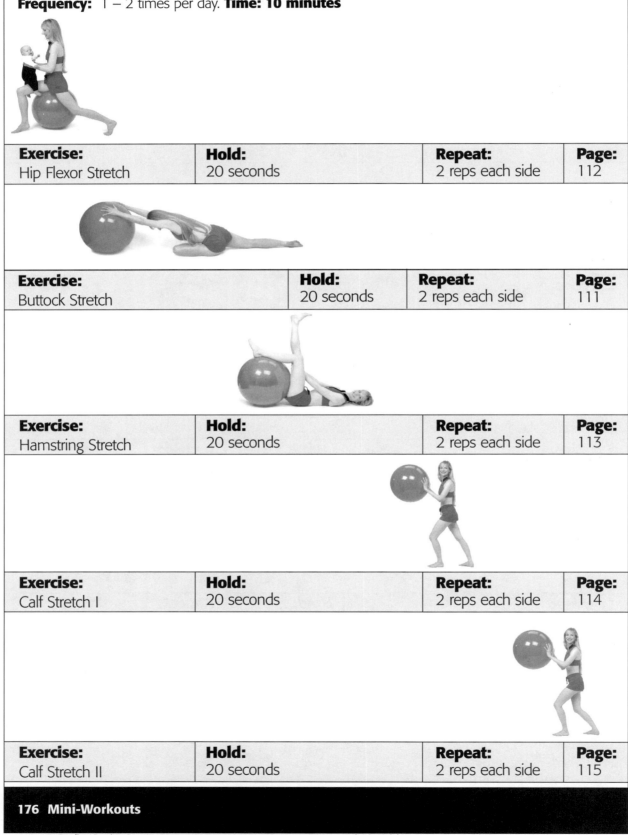

Exercise: Hip Flexor Stretch	Hold: 20 seconds	Repeat: 2 reps each side	Page: 112

Exercise: Buttock Stretch	Hold: 20 seconds	Repeat: 2 reps each side	Page: 111

Exercise: Hamstring Stretch	Hold: 20 seconds	Repeat: 2 reps each side	Page: 113

Exercise: Calf Stretch I	Hold: 20 seconds	Repeat: 2 reps each side	Page: 114

Exercise: Calf Stretch II	Hold: 20 seconds	Repeat: 2 reps each side	Page: 115

★★☆☆☆   Arm, Chest, and Upper Back Superset Workout

The following strengthening program is designed using the superset exercise technique. This exercise program is designed **without a rest break** between exercises. **Frequency:** 1 – 2 times per day, 2 – 4 times per week. After you become proficient with the workout below, increase to two sets of each exercise. **Time: 6 minutes**

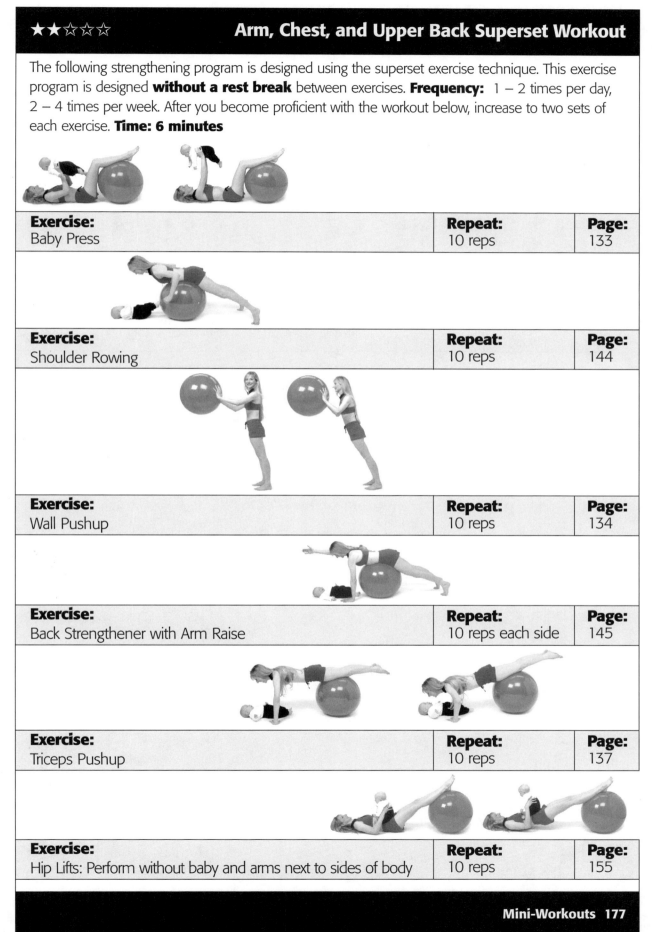

Exercise: Baby Press	**Repeat:** 10 reps	**Page:** 133

Exercise: Shoulder Rowing	**Repeat:** 10 reps	**Page:** 144

Exercise: Wall Pushup	**Repeat:** 10 reps	**Page:** 134

Exercise: Back Strengthener with Arm Raise	**Repeat:** 10 reps each side	**Page:** 145

Exercise: Triceps Pushup	**Repeat:** 10 reps	**Page:** 137

Exercise: Hip Lifts: Perform without baby and arms next to sides of body	**Repeat:** 10 reps	**Page:** 155

Abdomen and Back Superset Workout ★★★☆☆

The following strengthening program is designed using the superset exercise technique. This exercise program is designed **without a rest break** between exercises. **Frequency:** 1– 2 times per day, 2 – 4 times per week. After you become proficient with the workout below, increase to two sets of each exercise. **Time: 8 minutes**

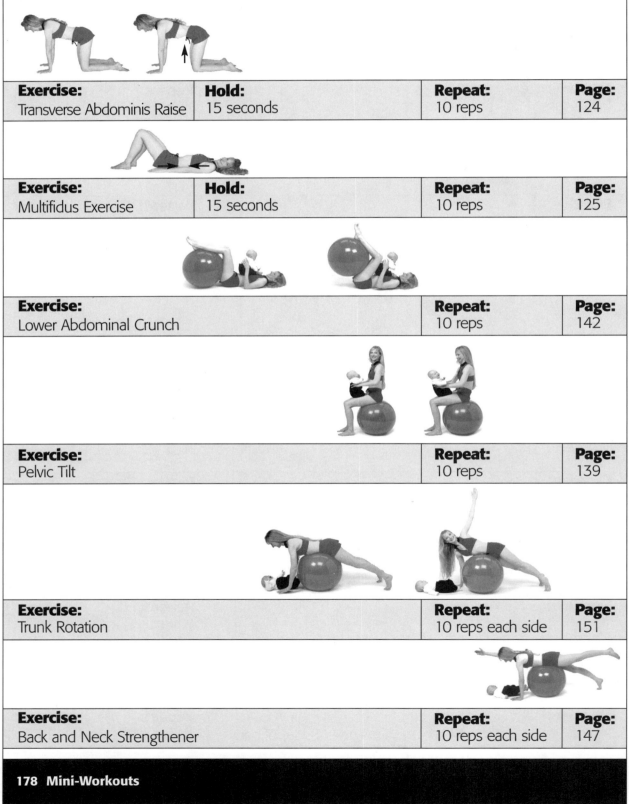

Exercise: Transverse Abdominis Raise	Hold: 15 seconds	Repeat: 10 reps	Page: 124
Exercise: Multifidus Exercise	Hold: 15 seconds	Repeat: 10 reps	Page: 125
Exercise: Lower Abdominal Crunch		Repeat: 10 reps	Page: 142
Exercise: Pelvic Tilt		Repeat: 10 reps	Page: 139
Exercise: Trunk Rotation		Repeat: 10 reps each side	Page: 151
Exercise: Back and Neck Strengthener		Repeat: 10 reps each side	Page: 147

The following strengthening program is designed using the superset technique. This exercise program is designed **without a rest break** between exercises. **Frequency:** 1 – 2 times per day, 2 – 4 times per week. After you become proficient with the workout below, increase to two sets of each exercise.
Time: 5 minutes

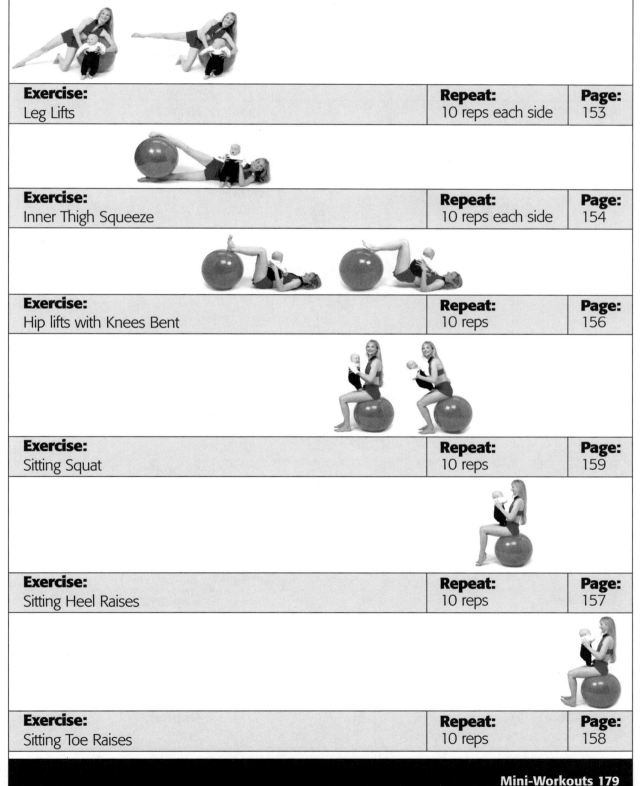

Exercise: Leg Lifts	**Repeat:** 10 reps each side	**Page:** 153

Exercise: Inner Thigh Squeeze	**Repeat:** 10 reps each side	**Page:** 154

Exercise: Hip lifts with Knees Bent	**Repeat:** 10 reps	**Page:** 156

Exercise: Sitting Squat	**Repeat:** 10 reps	**Page:** 159

Exercise: Sitting Heel Raises	**Repeat:** 10 reps	**Page:** 157

Exercise: Sitting Toe Raises	**Repeat:** 10 reps	**Page:** 158

The following strengthening program is designed using the compound exercise technique. This exercise program is designed **with a 20 second rest break** between each strengthening exercise. **Frequency:** 1 – 2 times per day, 2 – 4 times per week. After you become proficient with the workout below, increase to two sets of each strengthening exercise. **Time: 10 minutes**

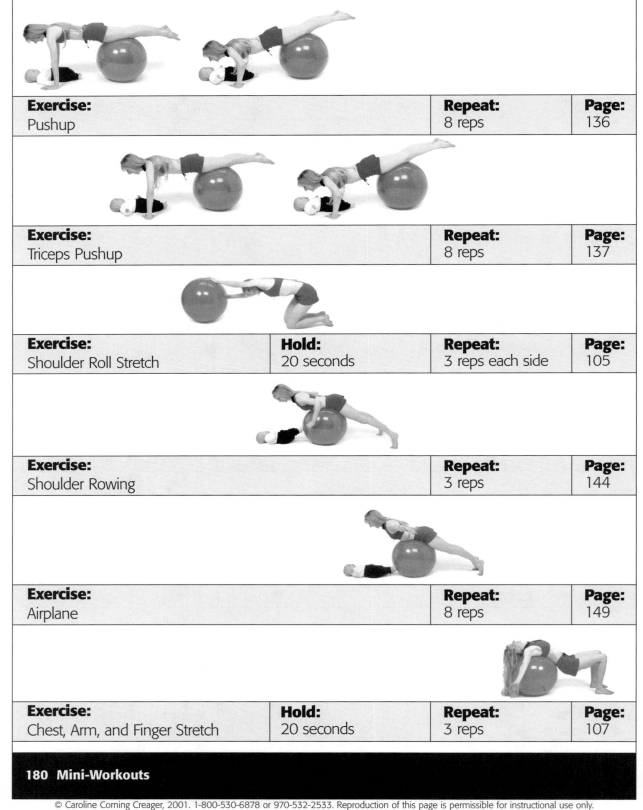

Exercise:		Repeat:	Page:
Pushup		8 reps	136

Exercise:		Repeat:	Page:
Triceps Pushup		8 reps	137

Exercise:	Hold:	Repeat:	Page:
Shoulder Roll Stretch	20 seconds	3 reps each side	105

Exercise:		Repeat:	Page:
Shoulder Rowing		3 reps	144

Exercise:		Repeat:	Page:
Airplane		8 reps	149

Exercise:	Hold:	Repeat:	Page:
Chest, Arm, and Finger Stretch	20 seconds	3 reps	107

The following strengthening program is designed using the compound exercise technique. This exercise program is designed **with a 20 second rest break** between each strengthening exercise.
Frequency: 1 – 2 times per day, 2 – 4 times per week. After you become proficient with the workout below, increase to two sets of each exercise. **Time:10 minutes**

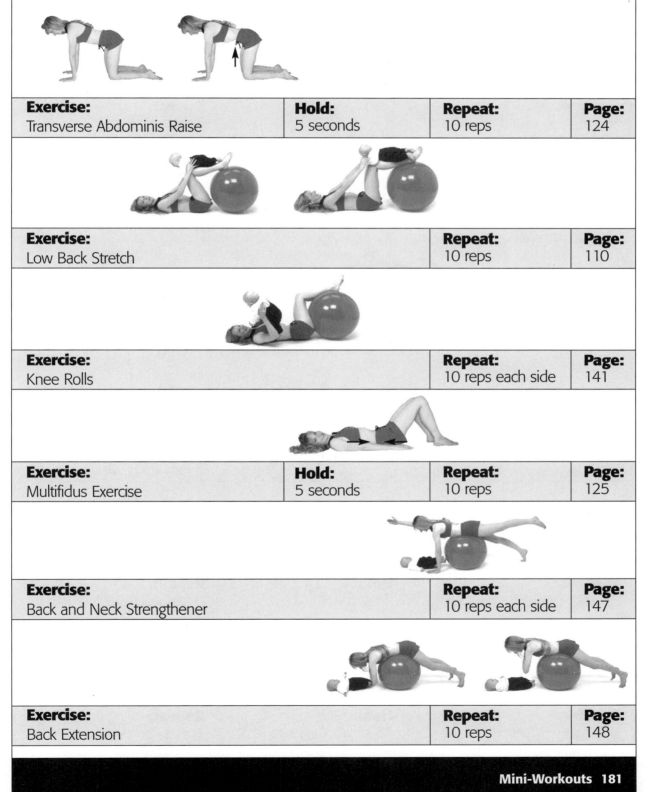

Exercise: Transverse Abdominis Raise	Hold: 5 seconds	Repeat: 10 reps	Page: 124

Exercise: Low Back Stretch		Repeat: 10 reps	Page: 110

Exercise: Knee Rolls		Repeat: 10 reps each side	Page: 141

Exercise: Multifidus Exercise	Hold: 5 seconds	Repeat: 10 reps	Page: 125

Exercise: Back and Neck Strengthener		Repeat: 10 reps each side	Page: 147

Exercise: Back Extension		Repeat: 10 reps	Page: 148

Abdomen Compound Workout

★★★★☆

The following strengthening program is designed using the compound exercise technique. This exercise program is designed **with a 20 second rest break** between each strengthening exercise. **Frequency:** 1 – 2 times per day, 2 – 4 times per week. After you become proficient with the workout below, increase to two sets of each strengthening exercise. **Time: 10 minutes**

Exercise: Lower Abdominal Crunch		**Repeat:** 8 reps	**Page:** 142

Exercise: Oblique Crunch		**Repeat:** 8 reps each side	**Page:** 143

Exercise: Abdominal and Back Stretch	**Hold:** 20 seconds	**Repeat:** 3 reps	**Page:** 108

Exercise: Trunk Rotation		**Repeat:** 8 reps each side	**Page:** 151

Exercise: Tummy Trimmin' Trunk Curl	**Hold:** 10 seconds	**Repeat:** 8 reps each side	**Page:** 152

Exercise: Side Stretch	**Hold:** 15 seconds each side	**Repeat:** 3 reps each side	**Page:** 109

The following strengthening program is designed using the compound exercise technique. This exercise program is designed **with 20 second rest break** between each strengthening exercise. **Frequency:** 1 – 2 times per day, 2 – 4 times per week. After you become proficient with the workout below, increase to two sets of each strengthening exercise. **Time: 10 minutes**

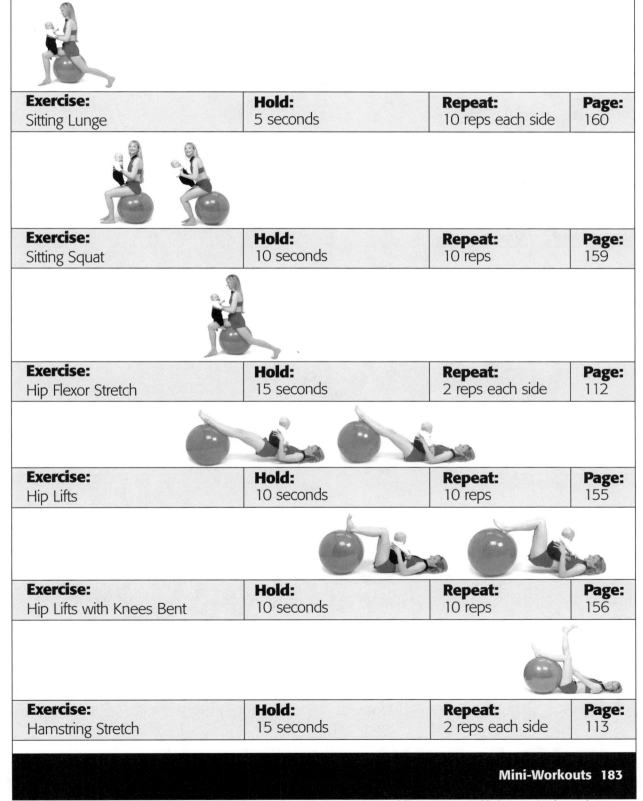

Exercise:	**Hold:**	**Repeat:**	**Page:**
Sitting Lunge	5 seconds	10 reps each side	160

Exercise:	**Hold:**	**Repeat:**	**Page:**
Sitting Squat	10 seconds	10 reps	159

Exercise:	**Hold:**	**Repeat:**	**Page:**
Hip Flexor Stretch	15 seconds	2 reps each side	112

Exercise:	**Hold:**	**Repeat:**	**Page:**
Hip Lifts	10 seconds	10 reps	155

Exercise:	**Hold:**	**Repeat:**	**Page:**
Hip Lifts with Knees Bent	10 seconds	10 reps	156

Exercise:	**Hold:**	**Repeat:**	**Page:**
Hamstring Stretch	15 seconds	2 reps each side	113

Legs Pre-exhaust Workout   ★★★★☆

The following strengthening program is designed using the pre-exhaust exercise technique. This exercise program is designed **with 20 second rest break** between each exercise. **Frequency:** 1 – 2 times per day, 2 – 4 times per week. After you become proficient with the workout below, increase to two sets of each exercise. **Time: 5 minutes**

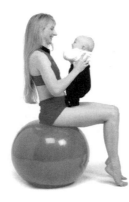

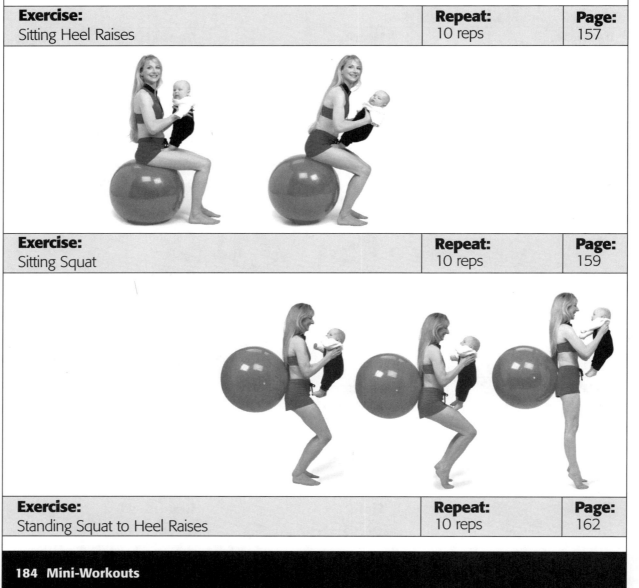

Exercise:	Repeat:	Page:
Sitting Heel Raises	10 reps	157

Exercise:	Repeat:	Page:
Sitting Squat	10 reps	159

Exercise:	Repeat:	Page:
Standing Squat to Heel Raises	10 reps	162

Glossary

Glossary

Anal sphincter: muscular rings that surround the anus and rectum.

Anus: a muscular opening at the end of the rectum.

Body mechanics: body positions used in activities of daily living to improve posture and lifting.

Bradycardia: an abnormally slow heart beat.

Cesarean delivery: delivery of a baby via the abdomen by a surgical incision.

Carpal tunnel syndrome: pain or numbness in the wrist, hand, or arm, caused by swelling and/or repetitive movements.

Collagen: a fibrous material found in the body; collagen fibers adhere together to form scar tissue.

Compound setting: entails exercising one muscle group with two different exercises, in an alternating manner.

Core muscles: the muscles that provide support and stability to your pelvis, spine, and abdomen.

Core stability: the ability of core muscles to control positional changes and return to their original position after being displaced.

Defecation: the act of having a bowel movement.

Diaphragm: is the largest and primary breathing muscle.

Diaphragmatic breathing: also known as belly breathing, is the correct form of breathing and is used during relaxation exercises.

Diastasis recti: separation of the rectus abdominis muscle from the midline of the abdomen.

Diastasis recti self-test: a simple test designed to ascertain the presence of a diastasis recti.

Episiotomy: a surgical incision made in the perineum to facilitate delivery of a baby.

Exercise ball: a round vinyl ball used for aerobic, stretching, and strengthening exercises. Also known as a Swiss Ball.

Exhale: breathe out.

External oblique muscle: mid-layer abdominal muscles, located on the sides of the abdomen, that assist with trunk rotation.

Exercise progression: a sequence of exercises.

Fast twitch muscle fibers: make up approximately 35% of the pelvic floor muscles, and are responsible for rapid and explosive muscle contractions yet short in duration, similar to a sprinter running a 100 meter dash.

Feces: stool, or body waste that is stored and released via the rectum.

Foam roller: a foam cylinder, or half-cylinder, used for stretching and strengthening exercises.

Friction massage: a massage technique used to breakup scar tissue adhesion.

Incontinence: an involuntary loss or accidental leakage of urine or feces.

Inhale: breathe in.

Internal oblique muscle: mid-layer abdominal muscles, located on the sides of abdomen (beneath the external oblique), that assist with trunk rotation.

Intra-abdominal pressure: pressure change that occurs within the abdomen. When you inhale, the diaphragm muscle contracts and moves down, compressing the abdominal contents and increasing (intra-abdominal) pressure on your bladder, bowel, and pelvic floor muscles.

Kegel: an exercise designed to strengthen your pelvic floor muscles, named after Dr. Arnold Kegel.

Kinesiotape®: a specialized tape used to break up scar tissue adhesion.

Log roll: a technique designed to decrease pressure and tension on an abdominal incision and the back, by rolling as a unit, from lying on the back to lying on the side.

Mediolateral episiotomy: a diagonal surgical incision made in the perineum, to the right or left of the anus, to facilitate delivery of a baby.

Midline episiotomy: a straight surgical incision made in the middle of the perineum to facilitate delivery of a baby. the most common type of episiotomy.

Mini-workout: an exercise routine.

Multifidus muscle: deep back muscles that work in unison with deep abdominal muscles to stabilize the spine.

Muscle substitution: using incorrect muscles to perform an exercise, as when fatigued.

Myofascial release: a form of manual therapy designed to break up scar tissue adhesion between the muscle and fascia.

Myotactic reflex: a reflex contraction that is triggered by bouncing or sudden stretching of a muscle, also known as a stretch reflex.

Neutral spine: a position where back is not arched or flat, it is somewhere in between.

Pelvic floor: muscles that support the pelvic organs, assist with sexual sensation, and sphincter control.

Perineum: the area between the vagina and rectum.

Perineum test: a test designed to assess pelvic floor muscle contractions by placing your fingers on the perineum.

Postpartum: after childbirth.

Pre-exhaustion: a technique used to focus on strengthening one muscle and follow it with an exercise that targets many muscles.

Pubic bone: a bone located in the pubic region. It attaches to the hip bones.

Quick Flick: an exercise designed to strengthen pelvic floor muscles and prevent urine leaking when coughing, sneezing, jumping etc.

Rectus abdominis muscle: a long muscle located in the middle of the abdomen, aka the "six pack muscle". It often separates during pregnancy.

Repetitions: the number of times an exercise is repeated.

Rest: a brief period that allows your muscles time to recuperate for the next set or exercise.

Resistive exercise: a form of exercise that utilizes resistance, such as ball exercises or free-weights, to improve strength.

Scar tissue adhesion: thickened scar tissue that occurs beneath the visible portion of the scar. May feel like a lump, and be sensitive to touch.

Scar desensitization: a massage technique used to make scar tissue less sensitive.

Scar tissue taping: a new technique used to break up scar tissue by applying specialized tape (Kinesiotape®) to gently stretch a scar.

Set: a number of repetitions performed in sequence without stopping.

Skin plucking: a massage technique used to break up scar tissue adhesion by lifting the scar away from body and moving it side to side.

Slow twitch muscle fibers: comprise approximately 65% of the pelvic floor muscles, account for slow twitch muscle contractions, and are required for endurance activities, such as standing throughout the day, or running a marathon.

Sphincter muscles: muscular rings that surround the anus, rectum, and urethra. They control the flow of urine out of the urethra and passage of stool from the rectum.

Start-Stop Tinkle Test: a test used to identify the ability to start and stop urine flow.

Stretch reflex: a reflex contraction that is triggered by bouncing or sudden stretching of a muscle, also known as a myotactic reflex.

Supersetting: exercising two opposing body parts with a minimal rest break between exercises.

Tail bone: a small bone at the base of the spine, also known as the coccyx bone.

Target area: a specified area of the body identified for a purpose, such as weak abdominal muscles identified for strength training.

Target heart rate: an age specific heart rate that determines individual exercise intensity.

Thoracic outlet syndrome: a condition caused by the compression of the nerves or vessels in the neck or armpit region, causing pain or numbness in the hands, arms, or neck.

Transverse abdominis muscles: deep corset-like abdominal muscles located on the side and front of the abdomen.

Trigger point massage: a massage technique used to break up scar tissue adhesion by applying gentle steady pressure to a small lump of scar tissue.

Ultrasound: a piece of equipment, used by physical therapists, that uses thermal effects to weaken scar tissue.

Urethra: the tube that carries urine from the bladder down to an opening in front of the vagina.

Urine: fluid waste excreted by the kidneys, stored in the bladder, and released via the urethra.

Vaginal self exam: a test designed to assess pelvic floor muscle contractions by placing the fingers in the vagina.

Visceral manipulation: a form of manual therapy designed to break up scar tissue adhesion located deep within the abdominal cavity.

References

Agency for Health Care Policy and Research, Public Health Service, U.S. Department of Health and Human Services. 1996. *Urinary Incontinence in Adults: Clinical Practice Guideline.* AHCPR Pub. No. 92-0038. Rockville, MD: Urinary Incontinence Guidelines Panel.

American College of Obstetricians and Gynecologists. 1994. Exercise during Pregnancy and the Postpartum Period. ACOG *Technical Bulletin 189.* Washington, DC: ACOG.

A.C.S.M. 1994. American College of Sports Medicine Position Stand: The Recommended Quantity and Quality of Exercise for Developing and Maintaining Cardiorespiratory and Muscular Fitness, and Flexibility in Healthy Adults. 1998. *Med Sci Sports Exerc.* 30(6): 975-91.

Anderson B., et. al. 1994. *Getting Into Shape: Workout Programs for Men & Women.* Bolinas, CA: Shelter Publications.

Baechle, T.R. 1994. *Essentials of Strength Training and Conditioning: National Strength and Conditioning Association.* Champaign, IL.: Human Kinetics.

Berg, H.C., Andersson, G.B., and Karlsson, K. 1991. Prevalence of Back Pain in Pregnancy. *Spine* 16(5): 549-52.

Bo, K. 2000. Pelvic Floor Muscle Exercise and Urinary Incontinence: Train Yourself Continent. *Tidsskr Nor Laegeforen* 120(29): 3583-9.

Bump, R., et. al. 1991. Assessment of Kegel Pelvic Muscle Exercises Performed after Brief Verbal Instruction. *Am J Obstet Gynecol* 165: 322-329.

Boissonnault, J., and Blaschak, M. 1988. Incidence of Diastasis Recti Abdominis during the Childbearing Year. *Phys Ther* 68(7): 1082-1086.

Clapp, J. 1998. *Exercising Through Your Pregnancy.* Champaign, IL: Human Kinetics.

Creager, C.C. 1994. *Caroline Creager's Airobic Ball Strengthening Workout.* Berthoud, CO: Executive Physical Therapy.

Creager, C.C. 1994. *Therapeutic Exercises Using the Swiss Ball.* Berthoud, CO: Executive Physical Therapy.

Creager, C.C. 1995. *Caroline Creager's Airobic Ball Stretching Workout.* Berthoud, CO: Executive Physical Therapy.

Creager, C.C. 1996. *Therapeutic Exercises Using Foam Rollers.* Berthoud, CO: Executive Physical Therapy.

Creager, C.C. 2001. Foam Rollers Facilitate Core Stability. *WorldWideSpine & Industrial Rehabilitation* 1(1): 16-19.

Cummings, G.S, and Reynolds, C.A. 1998. *Principles of Soft Tissue Extensibility and Joint Contracture Management.* La Crosse, WI: Orthopaedic Section, APTA.

de Leeuw, J.W., Struijk, P.C., Vierhout, M.E., and Wallenburg, HC. 2001. Risk Factors for Third Degree Perineal Ruptures during Delivery. BJOG 108(4): 383-7.

Eason, E., and Feldman, P. 2000. Much Ado about a Little Cut: Is Episiotomy Worthwhile? *Obstet Gyneco.* 95(4): 616-8.

Gerrits, D.D., Brand, R., and Gravenhorst, J.B. 1994. The Use of an Episiotomy in Relation to the Professional Education of the Delivery Attendant. *Eur J Obstet Gynecol Reprod Biol.* 56(2): 103-6.

Gilleard, W.L., and Brown, J.M. 1996. Structure and Function of the Abdominal Muscles in Primigravida Subjects During Pregnancy and the Immediate Postbirth Period. *Phys Ther.* 76(7): 750-62.

Guyton, A. 1987. *Human Physiology and Mechanism of Disease.* Philadelphia, PA: W.B. Saunders.

Hall, C., and Brody, L.T. 1998. *Therapeutic Exercises: Moving Toward Function.* Philadelphia, PA: Lippincott Williams & Wilkins.

Hides, J., et. al. 1994. Evidence of Lumbar Multifidus Muscle Wasting Ipsilateral to Symptoms in Patients with Acute/Subacute Low Back Pain. *Spine* (19)2: 165-172.

Hordnes, K. 1994. Episiotomy: An Appeal for a More Restricted Use. *Tidsskr Nor Laegeforen* 114(3): 3641-2.

Hulme, J. 1997. *Beyond Kegels*. Missoula, MT: Phoenix Publishing.

Kalkwarf, H. J., et. al. 1999. Effects of Calcium Supplementation on Calcium Homeostatsis and Bone Turnover in Lactating Women. *J Clin Endocrinol* Metab 84: 464-470.

Kotlyn, K.F., and Schultes, S.S. 1997. Psychological Effects of an Aerobic Exercise Session and a Rest Session Following Pregnancy. *J Sports Med Phys Fitness* 37(4): 28–91.

Labrecque, M. et. al. 1997. Association between Median Episiotomy and Severe Perineal Lacerations in Primiparous Women. *Can Med Assoc J* 15 156(6): 811–813.

Lindbolm, L.B. 1997. Exercise during Pregnancy. *Phys Sportsmed* 25(11): 28e-o.

Low, L.K., Seng, J.S., Murtland, T.L., and Oakley, D. 2000. Clinician-Specific Episiotomy Rates: Impact on Perineal Outcome. *J Midwifery Womens' Health* 45(2): 87-93.

MacArthur, C. et al. 2001. Obstetric Practice and Fecal Incontinence Three Months after Delivery. *BJOG* 108(7): 678-83.

Morved, S., and Bo, K. 1999. Prevalence of Urinary Incontinence During Pregnancy and Postpartum. *Int Urogynecol J Pelvic Floor Dysfunct* 10(6): 394-8.

Noble, E. 1995. *Essential Exercises of the Childbearing Year – 4th Edition*. Harwich, MA: New Life Images.

Ostgaard, H.C., and Anderson, G.B. 1991. Previous Back Pain and Risk of Developing Back Pain in a Future Pregnancy. *Spine* 16(4): 432-36.

Ostgaard, H.C., and Anderson, G.B. 1992. Postpartum Low-back Pain. *Spine* 17(1): 53-5.

Perez, P.G. 2001. An Overview of Medical Practice You May Encounter during Labor. *Lamaze Parents Magazine*. Spring/Summer, Pg. 52.

Prentice, A. 1994. Should Lactating Women Exercise? *Nutr Rev.* 52(10): 358-60.

Qian X, et.al. 2001. Evidence-based Obstetrics in Four Hospitals in China: An Observational Study to Explore Clinical Practice, Women's Preferences and Providers' Views. *BMC Pregnancy Childbirth* 1(1): 1.

Richardson, C., and Jull, G. 1995. Muscle Control – Pain Control: What Exercises Would You Prescribe? *Manual Therapy* 1: 2-10.

Richardson, C., Jull, G., Hodges, P., and Hides, J. 1999. *Therapeutic Exercise for Spinal Segmental Stabilization in Low Back Pain: Scientific Basis and Clinical Approach*. London: Churchill Livingstone.

Robinson, J.N., Norwitz, E.R., Cohen, A.P., Lieberman, E. 2000. Predictors of Episiotomy Use at First Spontaneous Vaginal Delivery. *Obstet Gynecol* 96(2): 214-8.

Samselle, C.M., et. al. 1999. Physical Activity and Postpartum Well-being. *J Obstet Gynecol Neonatal Nurs*. 28(1): 41-9.

Sapsford, R. 2001. Personal Communication.

Sapsford, R., Bullock-Saxton, J., and Markwell, S. 1998. *Women's Health: A Textbook for Physiotherapists*. London: WB Saunders Company.

Schwartz, M. 1987. *Biofeedback: A Practitioners Guide*. New York: Guilford Press.

Scott-Wright, A.O., Flanagan, T.M, and Wrona, R.M. 1999. C-Section Rates Higher Among Black than White College-Educated Women. *J Natl Med Assoc* 91(5): 273-277.

Shiono, P., Klebanoff, M.A, and Carey, J.C. 1990. Midline Episiotomies: More Harm than Good? *Obstet Gynecol* 76(3 Pt 1): 474-5.

Signorello, L.B., Harlow, B.L., Checkos, A.K., and Repke, J.T. 2001. Postpartum Sexual Functioning and Its Relationship to Perineal Trauma: A Retrospective Cohort Study of Primiparous Women. *Am J Obstet Gynecol* 184(5): 881-90.

Stephenson, R., and O'Connor, L. 2000. *Obstetric and Gynecologic Care in Physical Therapy*. Thorofare, NJ: Slack.

Shiono, P., Klebanoff, M.A., Carey, J.C. 1990. Midline Episiotomies: More Harm than Good? *Obstet Gynecol* 75(5): 765-70.

Smith, C. 1994. The Warm-up Procedure: To Stretch or Not to Stretch. A Brief Review. *J Ortho Sports Phys Ther* 19(1): 12-17.

United States Department of Health and Human Services. 1996. *Physical Activity and Health: A Report of the Surgeon General*. Atlanta, GA: U.S. Department of Health and Human Services, Centers for Disease Control and Prevention, National Center for Chronic Disease Prevention and Health Promotion.

Vera-Garcia, F.J., Grenier, S.G., and McGill, S.M. 2000. Abdominal Muscle Response During Curl-ups on Both Stable and Labile Surfaces. *Phys Ther* 80(6): 564-569.

Verhoef, M.J., and Love, E.J. 1994. Women and Exercise Participation: The Mixed Blessings of Motherhood. *Health Care Women Int* 15(4): 297-306.

Von Kries R., et. al. 1999. Breast feeding and Obesity: Cross Sectional Study. *BMJ* 319(7203): 147-50.

Webster's New World Dictionary: Second College Edition. 1982. New York: Simon and Schuster.

Wilder, E. 1993. *The Gynecological Manual: American Physical Therapy Association – Section of Women's Health*. Alexandria, Virginia: APTA.

Wilkes, J. 1999. *A Resource Guide for Incontinence and Stoma Care*. Montreal: Lieberman Press.

YMCA of the USA with Hanlon, T. 1995. *Fit for Two: The Official YMCA Prenatal Exercise Guide*. Champaign, IL: Human Kinetics.

Recommended Reading by Caroline C. Creager

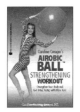

Caroline Creager's Airobic Ball Strengthening Workout by Caroline Corning Creager, ©1994; 64 pp. paperback; ISBN 0-9641153-1-X.

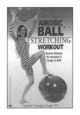

Caroline Creager's Airobic Ball Stretching Workout by Caroline Corning Creager, ©1995; 64 pp. paperback; ISBN 0-9641153-2-8.

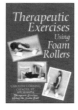

Therapeutic Exercises Using Foam Rollers by Caroline Corning Creager, ©1996; 236 pp. otabind paperback; ISBN 0-9641153-3-6.

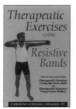

Therapeutic Exercises Using Resistive Bands by Caroline Corning Creager, ©1998; 366 pp. otabind paperback; ISBN 0-9641153-4-4.

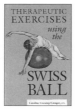

Therapeutic Exercises Using the Swiss Ball by Caroline Corning Creager, ©1994; 292 pp. otabind paperback; ISBN 0-9641153-0-1.

Ordering Information

To order Caroline Corning Creager's books, exercise balls, or foam rollers, please call one of the following distributors:

Australia/New Zealand:
Star Systems
61 (02) 6772 7433
www.starsystems.com.au

South Africa:
THERA MED
27 11 8046746
home.global.co.za/~dhtgo/

United Kingdom:
Osteopathic Supplies Limited
01432 263939
www.o-s-l.com

United States/Canada:
Orthopedic Physical Therapy Products
(800) 367-7393
(763) 553-0452
www.optp.com

To order Caroline Creager's books online, go to: www.amazon.com

To order *Women's Health: A Textbook for Physiotherapists* by Ruth Sapsford, et. al., contact Orthopedic Physical Therapy Products at the above number.

To order *Birth Ball: Use of Physical Therapy Balls in Maternity Care*, and *The Nurturing Touch at Birth: A Labor Support Handbook* by Polly Perez, contact Cutting Edge Press at (802)635-2142.

Index, continued

Index, continued